How Can You Eat That?

How Can You Eat That?

My journey into, through, and out of anorexia

Lily Johns

CHAPLIN BOOKS

www.chaplinbooks.co.uk

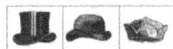

Chaplin Books
75b West St
Titchfield PO14 4DG
www.chaplinbooks.co.uk

I dedicate this book to my very dear friend
Emily C F Simms
who meant the world to me
and to so many others

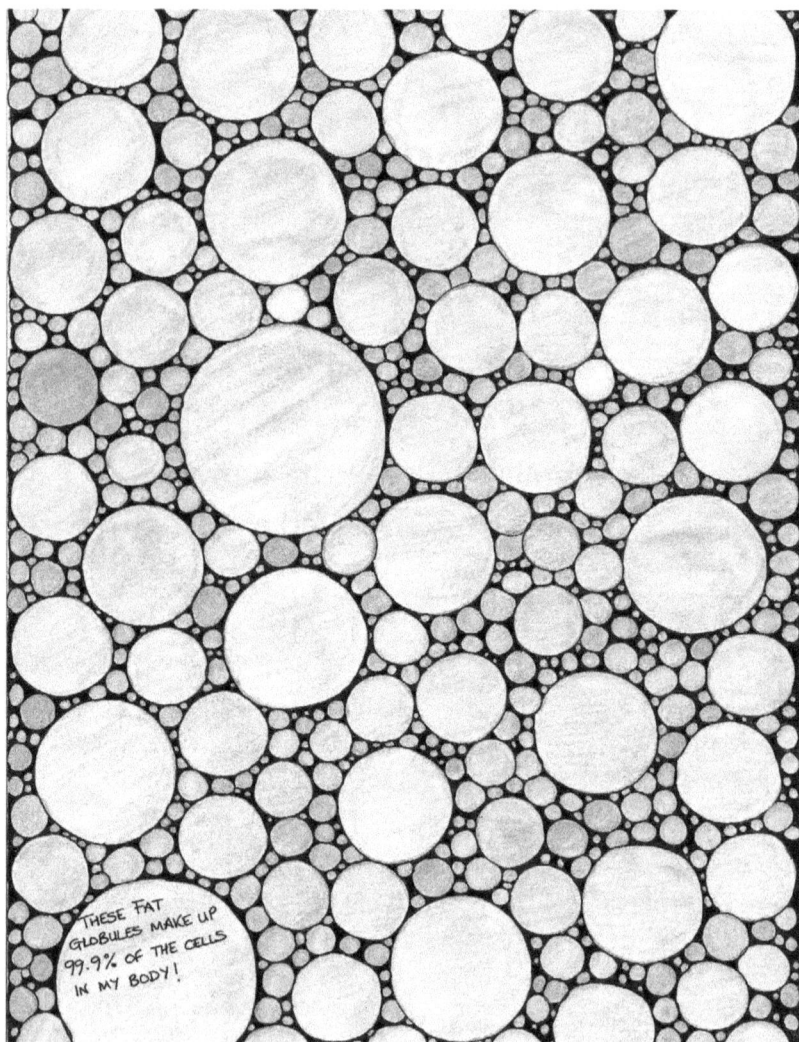

THESE FAT GLOBULES MAKE UP 99.9% OF THE CELLS IN MY BODY!

CONTENTS

Introduction

INTRODUCTION

I began my life as a confident, happy child but in my teenage years I started to suffer from lack of self-esteem and confidence. This developed into anorexia and depression which held me captive from my teenage years to my early 40s.

I am living proof that recovery from eating disorders is possible, but it is a tragic fact that all too frequently anorexics either die from their condition or stay an unhealthy weight for much of their lives. Even if a healthy weight is achieved, a sufferer can still possess an 'anorexic mind' and not be free of the negative thoughts that accompany the illness. In my early 40s I was certain I had fully recovered, but a three-year relapse in my late 40s showed me that this was not the case. Now I feel it's more realistic to speak about myself as being in remission from the illness.

During my long battle with anorexia, I rarely had any hope of being free and could never see a future for myself. I had such awful negative thoughts and found communication difficult, so I began to draw. I found drawing my thoughts not only gave me some kind of release from how I was feeling, but also allowed outsiders a peek into what I was going through. Some of those drawings are included in this book.

I also kept a diary. Now, years later, I am stunned - not only by how ill I had been, but also how desperate and misunderstood I had felt. Reading the diary has shown me how delusional I had been: what seemed to make perfect sense to me at the time I now see as evidence that I had lost all sense of reality. I realise now that my thinking was far too distorted and delusional for counselling to have had any chance of success. For much of the time I was too depressed to think rationally about what I was doing.

During those really bad times it meant a lot to have people not giving up on me, even though they didn't know how to help. During my illness I was never able to speak to someone who had recovered from anorexia, perhaps because so many never recover or perhaps because they do not wish to relive their experiences. It would have made a huge difference to me if I had known that recovery was achievable.

I have come to realise the importance of hope and how it is crucial for recovery. My boyfriend – later my husband - Tony was a constant support and always believed that I would get better from the illness. Completing an Alpha Course was also a turning point and from then on I believed that God would help me through the difficult times. I know that this might not be everyone's route to recovery, but coming to trust in God was paramount for me.

Some years ago, a dietician friend saw my drawings and felt that they could help people with anorexia or any other eating disorder: this motivated a deep desire in me to share my drawings and story. I also trust that my book will give parents, siblings, friends, partners, carers or nurses an insight into the thoughts and feelings that typically go through the 'anorexic mind'.

The people and places in this book have been anonymised to avoid embarrassment to my family and friends, hospital medical staff and adult mental health teams. My story, however, is one-hundred-percent true.

I have made every effort to minimalise potentially 'triggering' information and I would like to thank my dear friend Georgia for her insight and the feedback she gave me on this issue.

Lily John

CHAPTER 1

The Alien Beast

T ony, my boyfriend at the time, never gave up on me. He always believed I would get better. This is a letter he wrote early in my illness in the summer of 1997.

"My girlfriend Lily has a really pretty face. It is not just me that thinks so, but all my friends as well. I particularly love her nose, her lips, her eyes and her really soft skin. I also really like her gorgeous shoulders, great legs and great skin. There is not a part of her body that I do not love.

I was proud of her when we went out together. Although she felt uncomfortable, I liked her wearing high heels and short skirts to show off her great legs. I enjoyed knowing that my friends were jealous. I particularly liked a black dress, a brown suit and a beige raincoat. We did not necessarily agree on these, especially the black dress, but everyone who saw her in it said she looked gorgeous and she did. She looked a beautiful, sexy young woman and I was chuffed to bits to be with her.

My Aunt Jessie told me how the whole family thought how pretty she was and how nice she was. My mate Ian saw her at a weight-training course and told me "she's lovely – you'd best marry her!"

All the teachers at the school where I teach continually ask after her. They genuinely miss her. I think it is because one of her qualities is that she is a genuine person. She has compassion. She cares. She is honest. She would always do the little things that other people did not get round to doing. She was conscientious and hard-working and the students, especially those really close to her in her tutor group and basketball teams, loved her.

Her mother and father think the world of her, even though they may not always be able to show it. Her twin brother loves her to pieces and so does her sister.

My girlfriend has had a rough time. I know that better than anyone. Quite simply, she is fighting a battle to save her life. No battle could be harder than that. The whole world looks on in sympathy, some understanding more than others, but everyone willing her to win.

I know she does not realise what a nice, respected and good-looking person she is – how much she is appreciated and loved and how much she is missed. Perhaps when she does realise these things and accepts the opinions of others as fact and not fantasy, or even lies, she will take a huge step towards recovery.

We are told she will not be the same person again. She may not love who she loved before. She may not wish to do that what she did before. Things will change and there may be pain for others, and more pain for herself as she makes real-life decisions again, but what we want is for her to be in control of herself once again. We want her to be making decisions and not the alien beast which has taken her over and which is still controlling her now.

In recent days, I have seen glimpses of my girlfriend again. The alien has taken its first few knocks in years.

I say to myself everyday "keep fighting – you can do it." I wish I could fight for her. Perhaps in a very small way I am. She may find it difficult, knowing that I pray for her, but I do and I am not alone. I bet her family and other friends do too.

I am afraid that I took my girlfriend for granted. We drifted apart. I do not know if we will get together properly again when she is better. I really hope so, but we will have to wait and see. Whatever happens, I know she will always be someone I treasure and would trust with my life. I hope that she feels that way too – I know that she feels that way too.

One final thought. I have never felt that she would not make it. The light may seem a long way off for her now, but once she gets a glimpse of it, it will pull her towards it stronger and stronger until the darkness has gone and the alien has been destroyed. My girlfriend is a special person – she can do it. Trust me."

Tony

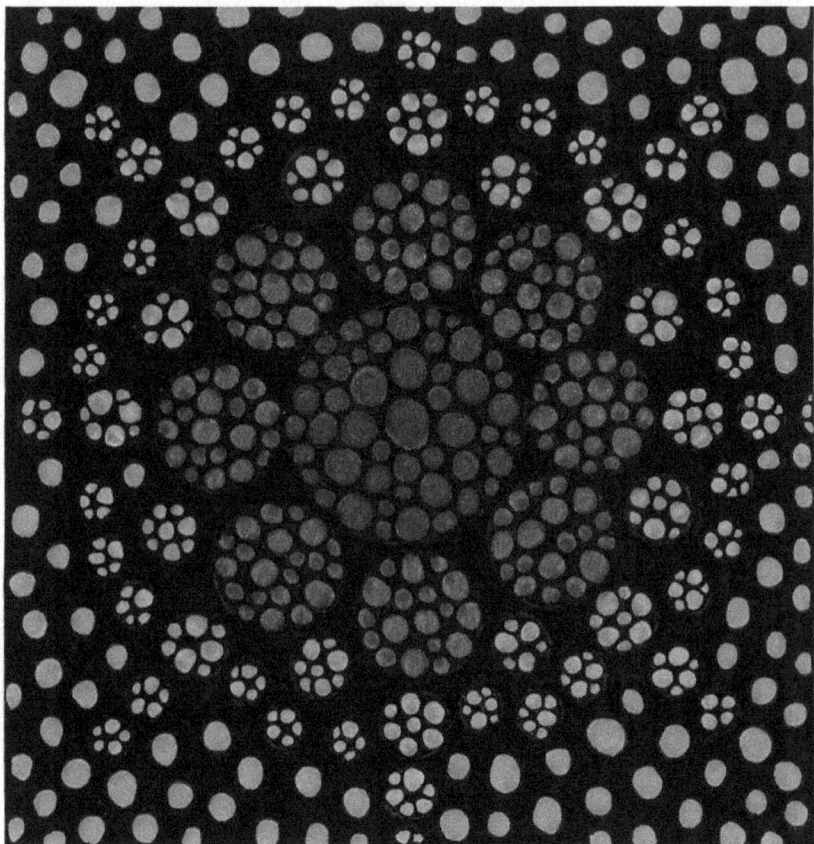

I feel like my head is going to explode

CHAPTER 2

How it All Began

L ooking back at photos of me, my twin brother James and my sister Helen playing in the garden and smiling, my childhood looked happy and idyllic. But I grew up thinking I was a very naughty child because I was always being told off. Mum would just shout at us, with the occasional smack if we had been really bad, but Dad scared the life out of me. His smacks would really hurt and sometimes I would be sent to my room for what seemed like hours. The time he most scared me was when he said that if I misbehaved he would hit me with the six-foot cane that had been delivered with a carpet a week or so before. I lived in dread of him doing that.

One day he came home from work late and heard about something naughty I had done during the day. I was just going to bed when he decided to tell me off. As I stood up, he shouted so loudly at me that the shock of it made me fall backwards onto the floor. I was terrified and ran off to bed, crying my eyes out. For once, Mum came to console me and was on my side saying that Dad really shouldn't have scared me in that way.

Looking back now, I can see we were brought up in a very disciplined way. We were taught that all adults should be respected and that they always knew best. When Mum and Dad had friends over, we were encouraged to only speak if they spoke to us: to be 'seen but not heard'. When I was told off, I always felt I was never given a chance to explain why I had done what I had - and even when I had done nothing wrong I was invariably not believed.

Sometimes we were told not to talk at mealtimes because we were taking too long to eat. Also if we didn't eat all our dinner, we would not be allowed pudding. As I loved my puddings, I remember sometimes feeling overly full because I had forced down all my dinner just so I could have that pudding.

We were never encouraged to talk about how we were feeling. On numerous occasions when I tried to explain how something made me feel - for example scared, nervous, or lacking confidence - I remember being told to 'stop being so stupid.' It was like emotions didn't exist. I certainly never remember Mum and Dad ever talking about how they felt about anything – it was never discussed; it was a case of 'keeping a stiff upper lip.'

I had been born in a Surrey hospital in 1968, just a few minutes before my twin brother James. I think Mum had quite a difficult pregnancy, hospitalised for some time due to very high blood pressure. She also had a caesarian section as one of our umbilical cords was wrapped around the other's neck. Life in the early days must have been difficult for my parents as my sister Helen was only eleven months older than James and me.

My first school was not far from where we lived, so every morning Mum would walk us there and then collect us again in the afternoon. I really enjoyed this school, had lots of friends and liked all the teachers. I always ran around in the playground playing games and had scraped and scratched knees on a daily basis, which required regular visits to the school nurse for plasters.

The only time I remember feeling unhappy at this school was when my brother and sister went to hospital to have their tonsils out, but I had to still go to school. In those days you had to stay in hospital for a couple of days after having your tonsils out, with a week or so at home to recover before being allowed back to school. I remember feeling hard done-by that my brother and sister didn't have to go to school, but I did and so most mornings I cried.

At the age of eight it was time to move on to our next school, which was a Middle rather than Junior School. It was then that Mum decided to get a full -time job as we were now old enough to walk home from school on our own. After we got home it would be a couple of hours before Mum would get home from work, so we became 'Latchkey Kids'. Helen, James and I were all pretty good at occupying ourselves in our garden or in the local park. As we were all born within eleven months of each other, we always had someone to play with and although there was the usual sibling rivalry, on the whole we did not get on too badly.

During that time, I can't remember Dad being around that much because by the time he came home from work, we were just going to bed. I do remember him having every other Sunday off. On this day he would take the three of us swimming, which we all enjoyed tremendously. However, while teaching us to swim, he did something that terrified me. He would lead us out to the middle of the pool and then let go - so we had no choice but to sink or swim. He was far enough away for me not to be able to reach him, but he could reach us (or so he said). I remember being frightened I was going to drown when he did this.

I was pretty happy at school. I remember being a confident child with no major worries. I would climb trees that were high and dangerous without a fear in the world. When, on a couple of occasions, I did come a cropper by falling out of one, I simply got up and tried again; nothing scared or fazed me.

Nearly all my friends were boys and I would play football with them in the playground at lunchtimes. I was beginning to show a talent for all kinds of sports and so the boys would always choose me first when picking teams. Mum was constantly moaning at me saying "Why do you have to play football? You are such a tomboy." I could never understand why a girl couldn't play football if a boy could, especially as I was as good as the boys. Why did I have to behave like a 'girl' was supposed to behave?

I got my first boyfriend when I was nine. We used to kiss in between the games sheds at break-times and I became very fond of him. I was devastated when one day he told me he was moving to Liverpool so I would never see him again. I vividly remember hiding under the table in our lounge at home in floods of tears for hours.

I had a teacher who had absolutely no control of the class. She was a lovely person, but some kids continually made her life hell. I remember one day being rude to her because I thought my friends would think I was cool if I behaved in the same way as they did. However, it backfired on me; she burst into tears and ran out of the class. I think my comment was the final straw for her and to this day I still feel so guilty about making her cry.

A group of boys with whom I was friendly decided one lunchtime to have a cigarette around the back of the school. I went with them, not because I had any intention of smoking, but just because they were my friends. For some reason one of them asked me to hold their cigarette for a few seconds … and at that moment a teacher caught me red-handed and we were all marched off to have a good talking-to by the Headteacher followed by our parents being informed. I was terrified about this because, even though I was innocent, I felt they would not believe me. I was constantly being told, or overhearing Mum say, that I was so easily led and had got in with the wrong crowd.

My friends always seemed to have money to buy sweets before and after school. This miffed me as I loved sweets but was never allowed to buy them as often as I wanted: only on Mum and Dad's terms. So one day, again feeling cross about this injustice, I took a small amount of money out of Mum's purse so I could spend it on sweets the following morning on the way to school. This stealing became a habit and continued for a couple of months. I knew that what I was doing was wrong and I was constantly terrified I was going to be found out. Our local sweet shop, unfortunately for me, was owned by our next-door neighbour and he soon cottoned on to what was happening and spoke to my Dad about his concerns. The next day a policeman turned up at our house and gave me a severe talking to. If that wasn't scary enough, both he and Dad told me that if I carried on the way I was, I would end up being sent to a juvenile detention centre. From that moment on, I was terrified that every time I misbehaved I might be imprisoned in the detention centre. Years later I learnt that Dad had known the policeman quite well and had secretly arranged for him to come down on me like a ton of bricks so that the shock treatment ensured I would be too scared to ever steal again. Their plan certainly worked as I was petrified for years to come.

Following this incident, I carried around an enormous burden of guilt and felt - right up to my thirties - that I must have been an incredibly naughty child. It wasn't until I mentioned to Mum and Dad how guilty I felt that they told me stealing from parents was very common in childhood. If they knew it was a normal childhood thing to do, why had they traumatised me at the age of ten? As Mum was constantly saying that I was easily led, she may have thought my friends were egging me on to steal this money and this was what persuaded Mum and Dad to keep me – and my brother and sister - away from the local comprehensive school and instead send us to a private school.

Once this decision was made, we were told that we had to start preparing for entrance exams: this involved Dad setting us homework before he went to work so that our English and Maths would be up to scratch. I wanted to go to the same school that Helen had gone to the year before but was told that I would not pass the entrance exam. As James was going to a boys' school, the search to find me an appropriate one began. I then wanted to go to the next-closest private school but was told that I would have to pass the Eleven Plus to get in, which I wouldn't be able to do. I remember being puzzled about why I wasn't even allowed to try, but there seemed no point in arguing. Perhaps Mum and Dad thought they were doing the right thing in not putting me through the exam which I would obviously fail and so would not have to suffer the disappointment.

They found a girls' convent school for me that would, in the words of my Mum, "take girls who couldn't get into other private schools." I still had to take an entrance exam and felt nervous and pressured about whether I would be accepted: the last thing I wanted was to fail to get into a school that took all those who couldn't get into other private schools! To everyone's relief, I did get accepted, and so I started my first day at a school miles from home without knowing a single person.

Dad used to take us all to school in the morning, doing a round trip in the car of about forty-five minutes before going on to work himself. Helen would get dropped off first, followed by James and then finally me. We all made our own way home, which involved me getting two buses and invariably that meant I didn't get home until 6pm. As I got older, if the second bus failed to turn up, I would walk the last two or three miles home.

Initially, I liked my school and made one or two close friends. However, I very rarely saw them outside school because of living so far away. I remember feeling jealous that my friends went around each others' houses after school and at weekends; something I was rarely able to do.

I soon shone in sports at school. The sport I was best at was hockey, mainly because I had joined a club at the age of eleven, but I was always one of the best in all the sports I tried apart from gymnastics and dance, which were not my forte. Our school had an indoor swimming pool, so I always swam at lunchtimes. I was always being told by my parents that what I lacked in academic achievement, I made up for in sporting success. The problem was, I didn't believe them. I always knew that Mum and Dad's main emphasis was on academic achievements: the importance of gaining the best exam results was constantly drummed into us. So I really didn't buy it when they tried to convince me that sporting success was just as worthwhile.

During my penultimate year at this school, when I was fourteen or fifteen, I became extremely unhappy. The main reason for this was that I was being picked on for being "too good at sport". Girls of this age can be horrible to be around and they were really bitchy to me. Sport, the only area I was succeeding in, suddenly became a bad thing and all I wanted to do was leave the school. Mum and Dad were aware of this and did look at a 'good' comprehensive girls' school in a different area (again, miles away from home) but it was eventually decided that I would stay where I was as I only had one more year to get through. Things did improve: during this last year I joined a girls' five-a-side football team run by my friend's father. Mum hated me doing this and constantly moaned about why I had to play football. She also took a dislike to my friend's family, thinking them 'common'. However, I loved this family and felt so at home with them; they always seemed pleased to see me and treated me well.

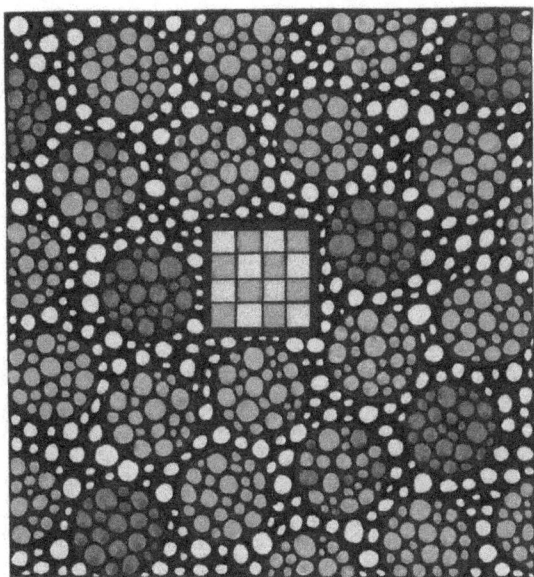

I feel so different to everyone else

Around this time I also had trials for the Middlesex County U16 Hockey Team and to my absolute delight got selected. I felt I had really achieved something and remember that this was one of the few occasions when my parents seemed genuinely proud of me. I went on to play for the U18 Middlesex team and then was part of the South of England squad. However, when I failed to be selected for the full England trial I gave up playing to this high standard. I have never been allowed to forget that by my Dad: he even mentioned this in his Father of the Bride speech at my wedding. But that's a different story, which I will come to later.

In 1984 it was time for me to take my O Levels (now called GCSEs). I was petrified I was going to fail them all because I knew I was no good at exams. I worked so hard revising every day, sometimes for eight hours a day, but got myself into more and more of a state. I ended up with four grade C passes, compared to James' and Helen's eleven or twelve A and Bs. I felt a complete dunce but kept being told by Mum and Dad: "never mind you tried your best, that's all we can ask."

I had a very close friend who I thought the world of, but the problem was that she was staying on to the Sixth Form in order to do A Levels, but I wasn't allowed to. My parents said the only subject on offer were too academic for me and I'd do much better going to the local Sixth Form College where I could do more obscure subjects such as the 'ologies'. So, much to my disapproval, I left school and my best friend after my O Levels at the age of 16. With some persuasion from Mum and Dad, I decided the two A levels to study would be Social Biology and Sociology, with CSEs in Physical Education and Health Science.

I very quickly settled into college life and enjoyed the new freedom of only having to be there when I had lessons. I had also started smoking a few months before, so being allowed to smoke on the college grounds was an exciting novelty. I suppose it was rather surprising that I started smoking as I was such a keen sportswoman, but it was just what most people did at that age. With my part-time job working in a supermarket, I was able to fund cigarettes and soon became a habitual smoker.

Helen was now attending the same school as James because it had a mixed Sixth Form. Although I was happy at my own college I did find that the conversations at home centred around their school and as I didn't know their teachers and the other pupils they constantly talked about, I felt very left out.

Whereas my childhood friends had been boys, I found it very difficult to talk to boys when I first went to college: many of them looked to me like grown men. Every time I talked to them I could not do it without blushing. Gradually I became a little more confident and ended up having lots of friends during my college days. I soon became fully involved in all the sports that the college offered and thrived on the fact that I could try sports I had never played before, such as basketball and squash. Soon I was in the college teams for every sport that I played and was rapidly becoming known as the best sportswoman at college. However, it was in my first year - at the age of 16 - that I became increasingly aware of the way I dressed and the way I looked; I was concerned what others thought of my shape and started to feel self-conscious. My success at sport increased my self-esteem but did nothing to stop these feelings of me not liking my body.

Sport was taking over my life and frequently I would miss lessons to play at the squash courts. Sport was really all I was interested in and during this first year I decided I would like to train to be a PE teacher. I didn't really fancy the teaching side of it, but I thought it was the only thing I could do in Higher Education that would allow me to carry on participating in sport all day and every day. I started working towards obtaining two passes at A level. I knew I wouldn't be able to get a place at one of the top universities like Loughborough, so it was suggested I look around for what were then called Colleges of Higher Education. In my second year of A levels I went to a number of interviews and ended up getting a place at a college on the South coast, on the condition that I obtained two

'E' grades or above in my A levels. I loved the feel of the place and was over the moon that I had been given a conditional place.

During my second year at college, I was doing so much sport that I developed a bad shoulder injury that stopped me from taking part in all the sports I wanted to. I couldn't play my beloved basketball and whenever I did play, for example squash, my shoulder would swell up and become painful. I started to worry about how I would cope with the practical side of my teacher training.

When I took my A levels in the summer of 1986 I gained one grade E pass in Sociology but an unclassified U in Social Biology. I am sure this was because I had missed so many lessons by choosing instead to play squash. This meant I had to retake Social Biology, spending another year at Sixth Form College, but fortunately the Teacher Training College kept my place open for a further year. This turned out to be a real blessing as it gave me another year to get my shoulder back to full strength. One thing that pleased me greatly was that James also ended up having to retake his exams because he didn't get the grades he needed to go to his choice of university. So, although unlike me he did not fail, it still meant that he and I would be at home at the same time.

During my final year at Sixth Form College I went through a really bad patch with Mum. It seemed that every day we would have full-blown arguments and end up yelling at each other. I was unhappy living at home. I think I felt I was old enough to do what I wanted, but was rarely allowed to do so.

Two years earlier, James had persuaded me to join the Venture Scouts. He was already a Scout and was moving up to the Venture Scouts, so it seemed natural for me to join him. I told him I would try it for a couple of weeks then decide if I wanted to join. I was nervous about not knowing anyone, but at least I had the comfort of my brother by my side. I soon got to love it – not only did I make lots of new friends, which once again Mum disapproved of, but I also got the opportunity to try new activities such as abseiling, rock climbing, caving, archery, scuba diving, hiking and survival training. These were all activities that a keen sportswoman was bound to relish and I most certainly did.

I also became involved in the Scout band and learnt to play the side-drum, albeit quite badly. I remember feeling good about being a real part of something worthwhile, whereas before I had only felt that way in sports teams. James and I began to work towards our Queen's Scout Award, which was the equivalent of the Duke of Edinburgh Gold award. This enabled me to become a Beaver Scout leader and to be involved with expeditions in the Brecon Beacons and Lake District. Overall this was a happy time for me. I became very close to a family whose son was also in the Ventures. I called them my 'adopted parents' and James and I spent every opportunity we had around their house, although this did not please Mum. I always had good fun at their house, much more than I ever had in my own home. I always felt that I was being treated unfairly at home for either being told off for things I didn't do, or for not being able to do what I wanted.

During this time in the Venture Scouts we started getting into a hectic social life with numerous parties, discos and weekends away. This was at the time when I was so concerned with how I looked. I would take ages to decide what to put on for the discos and often changed outfits five or six times, never feeling that I looked good in any of them. I remember standing in front of the full-length mirror in Mum and Dad's room and asking Mum over and over again whether my bum looked big in what I was wearing. She would always respond in the same way saying: "For goodness sake don't be so stupid … look you've just inherited my pear shape!" This distressed me as I thought my Mum was quite big in the thighs and bottom. She might as well have said: "You look the same as I do". I can now see that I was never anything like her shape, but her comments made me believe I was.

In the summer of 1987, I finally achieved my A level pass in Social Biology, which meant I could go off to Teacher Training

College. James also got his grades and was off to university to study Dentistry. I found the thought of leaving Sixth Form College difficult as I really did enjoy it there, but even though I was nervous of going to a new college I was relishing the thought of leaving home. I felt very much like I had outstayed my welcome there.

CHAPTER 3

Does Thinner Mean More Attractive?

For my first year at Teacher Training College, I stayed in the college campus' hall of residence. There were about a hundred rooms in the block so it was always very noisy, but probably a good place to get to know a lot of other students quickly.

It soon became clear to me that most girls on my course were quite masculine looking and some openly said they were gay. I began to feel insecure as I was concerned that the boys and lecturers might think I too was gay. I started to believe that if I wasn't thin, people would presume I was gay, so I became more self-conscious about my weight and how feminine I looked, especially as we spent nearly all our time in tracksuits. I had no prejudice against anyone gay: I just didn't want other people to think I was when I wasn't. This fear stemmed from being concerned with what others thought of me.

I enjoyed my course in the first year, especially the practical side. I didn't really embrace the social side of college life but worked hard on the academic side, which I invariably used as an excuse for not socialising. I didn't really feel part of a group when out in the evenings so instead locked myself away, where I felt more secure.

For the second year, we were no longer able to live on campus so with two friends – Zara and Hattie – I moved into a house about two miles from the college. This arrangement worked well to start with, but the house was grotty and damp and had no central heating, so it was always freezing cold. After the first term, Hattie wanted to leave the house so a girl called Vicki, who was on my course, took her place. She was gay and not afraid to tell anyone, so all my fears of others thinking I was also gay came flooding back.

Vicki had her gay friends around all the time. They were mainly men and very camp; I felt I had nothing in common with them. The only places in which they would socialise in the evenings were gay bars and clubs. Although I was often invited out with them, I felt uncomfortable in that environment, especially when they would snog their partners in front of me. So, once again I began to stay in most nights to avoid having to socialise, putting all my efforts into the assignments for which I was receiving top marks. This was something I had never experienced before; it gave me a massive high and spurred me on to continue to work even harder.

When the third year of my course started, I ended up with nowhere to live and asked Vicki if I could crash on her floor. I thought it would only be for a couple of weeks, but it ended up being for a whole term. The house was also a complete mess and really dirty, but I felt I couldn't do or say anything because I didn't officially live there. I spent the whole of the first term in my third year trying to find somewhere to live and people to share with. Eventually I found a nice house not far from the college and moved in with a sports science student and another lad who was on my course. It started off well, but I soon became aware that this lad was a drug dealer. There were always frequent knocks at the door with people coming round to buy their 'fixes' and I remember being constantly worried that we would be raided by the police, especially as he would leave his stash of drugs and weighing scales around the house in full view.

It was while I was living in this house that I decided to go on my first major diet. I was unhappy with the way I looked and was sick of always feeling self-conscious and lacking in confidence. The female students that I admired at college not only had bodies to die for, but also had countless boyfriends. I remember thinking that if I just lost some weight I would turn into an attractive, confident person that lads would fancy. I also thought this would encourage people to think I wasn't gay. I planned meticulously what I was going to eat. I ate once a day in the evening, mainly salad, a little bit of rice and a sprinkling of peanuts to give me energy; I couldn't risk feeling faint because my course was pretty energetic. Soon it became obvious that I was losing a fair amount of weight and people began to make comments. This simply spurred me on to make my diet even stricter and my main goal became to lose weight no matter how rubbish that made me feel. One of the lecturers spoke to my friend saying: "I'm worried about the weight Lily has lost – you don't think she's anorexic, do you"? However, nothing was ever said to me about their concerns and I was never sent to the college doctor or nurse. I therefore decided that I obviously hadn't lost enough weight as to be seen as 'skinny' (which is what I wanted to be), so I just kept plunging deeper and deeper into eating less and less.

The end of the third year came and I remember dreading going back to my parents for the summer holidays. I knew that if I didn't eat while I was with them it would cause endless rows and the atmosphere would be awful. So I decided to go to my parents and eat normally until I went back to college in September. However, I do remember skipping lunch everyday while I was at work at my temporary job at a local garage, a job I held for two years. It turned into the dream job for me as it meant that all day I was driving brand new cars and doing masses of overtime, which I didn't mind at all. More importantly, the people there were lovely and I felt at ease in their company. It was obvious that some of my male colleagues fancied me, so this also improved my self-esteem and confidence. A lot of people had commented on my weight loss when I first went back to my parents at the start of the holidays, but as I was now putting on some weight, I'm sure they thought that as a student I probably couldn't afford to eat, or was too busy partying to eat. Little did they know that the real truth: that I was already caught in the grips of the 'downward anorexic spiral'.

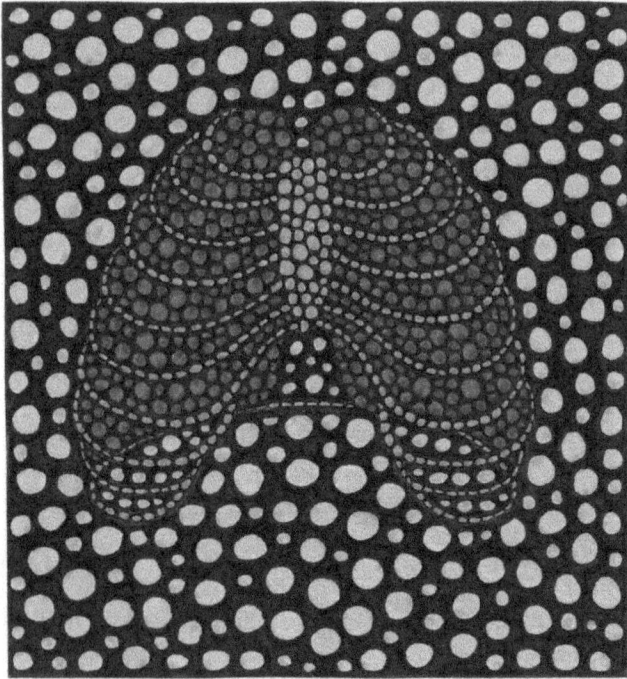

I just want to feel my ribs again

I was to live back on campus in my fourth year at college. We had a whole term of teaching practice on our return from the summer holidays, so I was really pleased about these new living arrangements. Our evening meals were provided by the college and were paid for as part of our rent. I was once again in complete control of my food intake. I was conscious of the fact that I had put on weight over the holidays and was very concerned that others would notice. From this time on, I had it all planned in terms of what I was going to eat. Most days during this first term back (during my teaching practice) I would have no breakfast and eat a few Ryvita for lunch. I would skip the cooked dinner provided by the college and have a salad and apple in the evening. I have no idea how I managed to survive that teaching practice on so little food, but I did and I also managed to obtain a really good grade. Nevertheless, I couldn't wait to finish the teaching practice, not just because it was really hard work, but because I could then restrict my food intake even further. The next two remaining terms were focused on finishing our dissertations and taking our final exams. There were very few lectures and no practicals, so I knew I could get away with eating less and less. If it happened that I did eat more than I had intended, I remember feeling angry, as if I'd let myself down. I soon became totally obsessed with what the scales said. My energy levels were at an all-time low, so really all I did in the second term was sit at my desk with my computer completing my dissertation. I worked all the hours I possibly could, using the fact that I had work to do as an excuse for not socialising, but also to take my mind off how hungry I was all the time.

After Easter all the final-year students had to start to think about applying for full time jobs as PE teachers, as well as finishing our dissertations and taking our final exams. I was unsure about whether I really wanted a teaching job, but after spending four years taking a degree in Physical Education felt I had no option but to apply. I thought that if I told my parents (after they had partly funded my degree) that I didn't want to teach after all, my life would not be worth living.

I began some research for my dissertation in a school watching mixed-sex basketball lessons. I went to this school on a number of occasions to do a video recording of the Head of Department teaching. I remember being astounded by what a good teacher he was, but also I began to realise that I fancied him, even though he was a fair bit older than me. However, I finished my research and didn't really think any more of it.

I applied for a teaching job at a school 40 miles from the college (I was adamant I didn't want to look for jobs back in my home town) and was offered an interview. Quite a few on my course had already got jobs and some had decided not to teach at all. There were very few of us at this time who were still looking for jobs. I think I hadn't really shown much interest in applying because I was still unsure whether I really wanted to teach and had therefore left it to the last minute. The day before my interview my lecturer received a phone call from the Head of Department at the school in which I had done my research, asking him whether he knew of any PE students who hadn't got a job yet, as there was a vacancy in his school. My lecturer, who I got on very well with, luckily thought of me and came round to my hall of residence to tell me to get to the school in two hours for an interview.

Before I knew it, I was at an interview at that school. I spent the morning being interviewed by the Head of PE and then the afternoon being interviewed by the Deputy Headteacher (as the Headteacher was on a course that day). When I got the job, which started in September, I was over the moon because not only was it known as one of the best schools in the area, but because I really liked the Head of PE.

So after contacting the first school in which I had been offered an interview to tell them I had accepted a post elsewhere, all I had to worry about was passing my dissertation and then my final exams. As always happens with me, I was panic-stricken about the exams, but fortunately they only counted for a third of my final marks. About three weeks after these exams I found out that I had been awarded a 2:1 degree: I was thrilled. I remember thinking "Fancy me, the non-academic one, getting the same degree grade as my sister and my brother." It showed, in my opinion, that what makes the difference to how well you do is how interested you are in what you are studying.

CHAPTER 4
How Can You Eat That?

In August 1991 I moved to a shared house with two other newly qualified teachers – one teaching science and the other music. This was such a nerve- wracking time because not only was I sharing a house with two people I didn't know, but this really was the start of proper adult life. I was also living in a completely new area where I knew no one – I didn't even know where the nearest shops were.

I started work at the beginning of September and soon got into the swing of things. It really helped that I got on well with Tony, my Head of Department. He was very approachable if I had any difficulties and was always willing to give helpful advice.

The following month, I had my graduation ceremony. Looking back at the photos of this day now, I can't believe how thin I was – my legs were like matchsticks. I don't think any other photos were taken of me those four years I was at college, so it was quite a shock for me to see how thin I was at that time.

There was so much to learn during my first year at the school and it was hard working full-time. However, I was enjoying it and my social life was improving. I especially remember Tony taking me and my two housemates out on some evenings to the local pubs. (Tony was on his own at that time, bringing up two very young boys). I soon realised that I really fancied him but was worried about the age gap of nineteen years. Once again, I was concerned what others would think. I also struggled to believe that he would ever be interested in me and was convinced that he fancied one of my housemates. Anyway, it got to the end of the first term and during the Christmas holidays I spent some time with Tony, with it soon becoming clear that there was a mutual attraction between us. We started dating on 22 December 1991 but decided to keep it to ourselves, not only because his boys were so young, but also because we didn't think it would look good at school. Little did we know that other people had guessed long before we made it public knowledge.

The next term went well. Tony had organised a school trip to America for the Easter holidays and, as I'd never been to America before, I asked if I could go too. That became our first holiday together (although we did have twelve schoolchildren with us). Looking back at photos from that time, I was an average size, so had obviously given up dieting at that stage. However, I still really lacked confidence and was always worried what others thought of me.

The summer term arrived and I had to have my final assessment from the County Inspector in order to pass my newly qualified year - fortunately I was successful. Teaching PE in the summer is supposed to be one the nicest parts of the job, but for me it was really difficult. All the other PE staff were wearing shorts or gym skirts with T-shirts or vest tops, but because I was so self-conscious I kept wrapped up; I couldn't bear to look at myself. Although I was eating normally during this year and had returned to a healthy weight, I never lost the feelings of self-hate and of being embarrassed by my body. By staying 'wrapped up', lots of questions and comments arose as to why I wasn't wearing the same as the others and I ended up drawing more attention to myself.

During that summer I bought my first house – a two-bedroom maisonette that ended up being my home until 2008.

Although, over the next four years I did my job well, there was always the underlying issue that even though I was a 'normal' weight, I felt self-conscious about my figure and always felt I looked fat and that I would be more attractive if I were slimmer.

A massive turning point in my life happened in 1995. I had always had a 'sweet tooth' and even though I felt guilty, every break-time I would go the canteen to buy a homemade biscuit or Chelsea bun. One day I was sitting in the staff room eating my Chelsea bun when a member of staff shouted out, so everyone could hear: "How can you eat those every day and not get huge?" Instead of taking this to mean that I was lucky I wasn't getting fat, which is what I am sure was intended, I took it to mean that unless I did something to stop this, I was going to get huge. As I felt huge already, I took the decision that from that moment on I would no longer eat sweet things and would begin a diet. I was devastated that this member of staff had given everyone the impression that I ate a Chelsea bun every day; I felt so ashamed. From that moment on it was the start of a very slippery slope for me, one from which it would take years to escape.

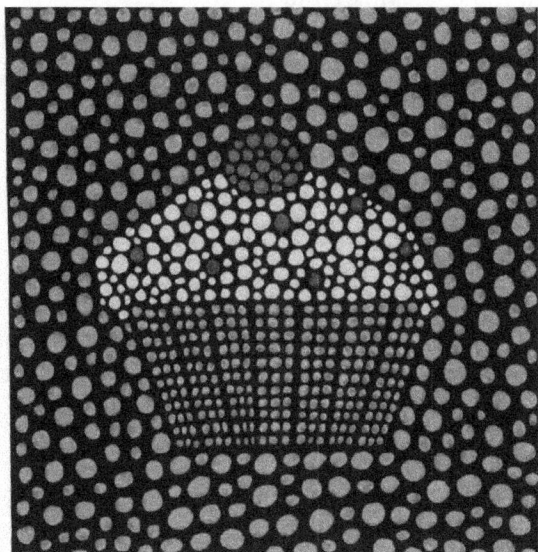

Why have I got such a sweet tooth?

From then on, my weight plummeted and in January 1996 I had to have six months off work because I was too ill to do my job. I remember Tony taking me to the doctor at the end of 1995 and her telling me that I had anorexia. I found this difficult to accept as I felt I was too big to be anorexic and, at twenty-seven, too old; I also liked food too much. I really didn't realise at that time how ill I was, but it soon became evident that I was too ill to work. I was referred by my GP to a Community Psychiatric Nurse and a dietician. I wasn't at all willing to be helped by these two professionals because I still found it difficult to accept that I was ill.

In June 1996 it was decided I would go back to work part-time, ready to start full-time again in September. My weight had increased during this time, though by June I was still a little underweight. I still found work difficult as I never seemed to have any energy. My mind was in so much turmoil with such negative and depressive thoughts, that I was constantly exhausted.

That summer Tony and I went on holiday to Spain to an apartment in Malaga. All we did for two weeks was lie by the pool and in the evenings go out to eat. I was hardly fat, but I remember really struggling to look at myself in a bikini and I just detested myself for eating a relatively normal diet. I knew I would live to regret what I was eating - which was, in fact, healthy salads and grilled meat - but I also knew that it was only for a short period of time until I was home and could starve myself again.

I went back to work full time in September and started seeing another dietician who I really liked and also a psychologist who I was much less keen on. I was signed up for sixteen sessions with the psychologist but it was a complete waste of time. She had the ability to make me feel really self-conscious and extremely uncomfortable; I just didn't gel with her at all. Quite often there would be long silences during which she just stared at me. One time there was a silence lasting almost an hour - the whole session - and I remember thinking that if she couldn't be bothered to talk to me then why should I bother to talk to her? Looking back, I am sure that this was a tactic of hers to get me to say something, but all it achieved was me disliking her even more and wondering why I was wasting my time seeing her. I was also depressed at that time and found communication difficult, so our sessions were always going to be doomed to failure.

My relationship with Tony wasn't going too well either. We were arguing a lot at work: he was caught in the middle of knowing that I wasn't well, but also needing to make sure that I was doing my job properly – which I wasn't. We also argued a lot about what I was doing to myself, which he thought was totally unnecessary. I will never forget what he said to me in December 1996. He asked me what was more important to me: our love for each other or my body image? The problem was, I couldn't answer him. I knew that there was nothing more important to me than losing weight and trying to be thinner. That became my number one priority over work, over my relationship with Tony, over my family, in fact over everything. The quest to lose weight had completely taken over my life.

In January 1997, I had a session with the psychologist during which we talked about fifteen styles of distorted thinking. I soon realised that I had 13 of those styles. She told me that my negative thoughts had developed over such a long time that they had totally blocked out all my positive thoughts.

To aid my weight loss I decided to step up my exercise routine: this turned out to be highly successful but resulted in me increasingly lacking energy. I remember a colleague one day asking me whether I was OK because I was looking very frail. This really pleased me as I thought I couldn't be fat if I looked frail. Another colleague asked whether swimming was the only exercise I did? I took this to mean that I should be doing more exercise, otherwise why would she ask unless she thought swimming wasn't enough? My thinking was getting so distorted – anything anyone said, I turned around so that the meaning was the opposite to the one intended.

Months before, I had stopped menstruating again so I knew I

was doing something right in my quest to lose weight. That still wasn't enough for me, though. My psychologist said that my thoughts and beliefs about myself were so deep-rooted that I found it very difficult to accept that they weren't true and therefore were very hard to challenge. She was trying to treat me using cognitive behavioural therapy, but it was just not working. That same session she said that my life was really unhappy and that this was sad.

Things got worse at work in February 1997. I felt people were out to get me big-time. I used to swim at a health club, which quite a few other members of staff attended and I felt that they were telling senior management at work every time they saw me there. Even at my step-aerobic classes at the local leisure centre, there were people that I knew from work. That same week the deputy head at work asked to have a meeting with me and gave me a really hard time. She said I lacked the enthusiasm I used to have with my tutor group and with my lessons. She also said that I was always sitting down and not interested anymore. I felt like the whole world was out to get me. I blamed Tony for telling other staff things about me that were none of their business, but his response was that they all cared about me. I would not accept this and continued to be very angry with him.

My depression continued to get worse. I really felt that I was fighting the illness all on my own with no one really caring: on the contrary, they were out to get me. Thoughts of suicide began to enter my head; it was really the only way out that I could see. I also felt the medical profession was letting me down by not getting me better and I even had awful thoughts that I wanted to punish them for not caring enough to get me better. My psychologist was also threatening not to treat me anymore as my weight was dropping. Even though I didn't mind not seeing her, for me it was just another example of someone giving up on me - and this was someone who was supposed to be the eating disorder specialist for my health authority.

In the Easter holidays of 1997, Tony and I once again travelled to America with one other colleague and a group of students for an eight-day stay in the Boston area. This was an awful time for me because staying with a host family meant I had to eat the food they cooked, or else appear rude and ungrateful. This left me feeling guilty and angry with myself - so angry that I took all my frustrations out on Tony. He in turn was angry with my attitude towards eating a normal amount of food. I was also unable to keep up my exercise routine and that too caused me a lot of grief. During this eight-day stay I put on five pounds. Why, I thought, is it so easy to gain weight but so hard to lose it? I returned from America determined to finish my relationship with Tony as I felt we just didn't get along any more and I also felt he no longer was on my side.

In that same month I decided to go along to an Eating Disorder Conference held at Guy's Hospital in London. Dad came with me as I was really worried about going, being convinced that I would be the fattest attending. To my surprise there were normal-weight people there and, as expected, lots of really thin people as well, but probably not as many as I had expected. There were a few women who were the thinnest I had ever seen, and although I felt physically sick looking at their incredibly skinny bodies, at the same time I felt jealous of the obvious control they had to restrict their food intake much more successfully than me. I so longed to have that kind of control.

Once again my weight dropped below a level I had been trying to achieve since going back to work the previous September. I realised the jubilation I felt and the buzz I experienced from achieving this meant I was back once again on the slippery slope, but I really didn't care because it made me feel so good.

When I met once again with my psychologist in May, she made it clear that I had to think of other things that made me feel better about myself. The problem I had was that nothing outside exercise or losing weight made me feel any better. I realise now how sad that was, but that was how I felt.

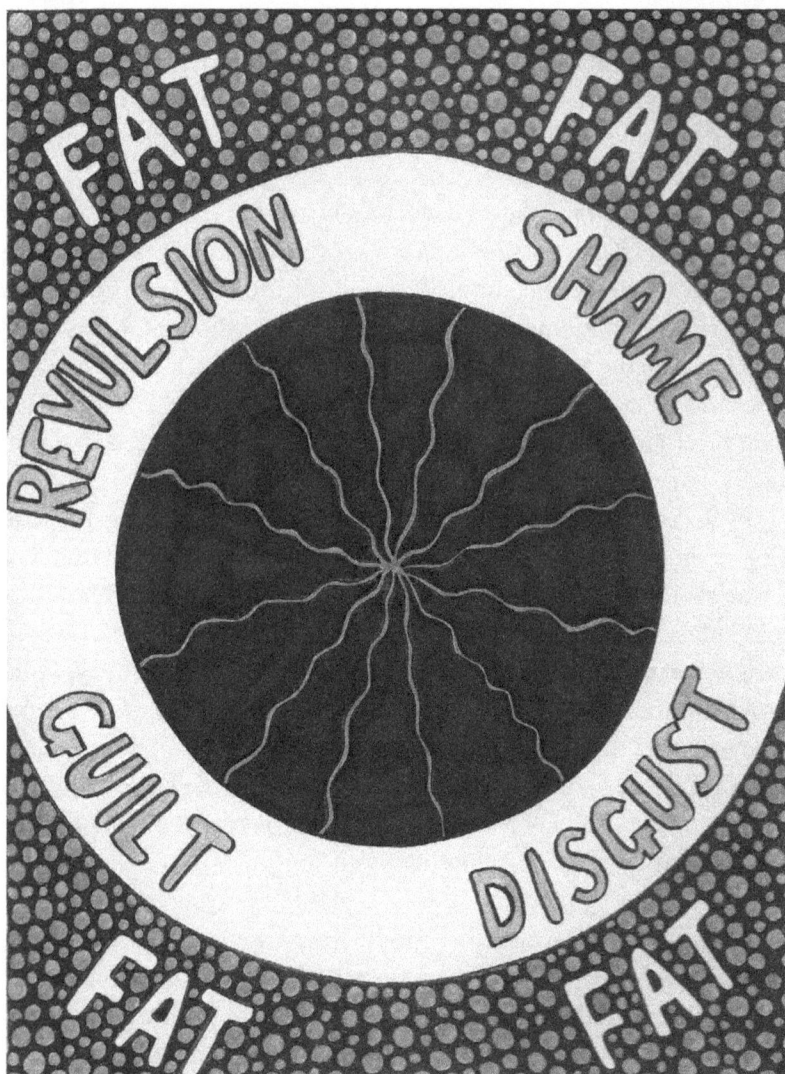

By the end of May I had lost more weight. I once again met with my psychologist, who admitted to me that she didn't know what to suggest anymore. According to her we were "pulling in opposite directions" and not only that but I had "gone into a cave and was not prepared to come out". She also said that I hadn't made the effort to change. So, at the beginning of June, she gave me an ultimatum – she didn't want to see me again until I was ready to change. She said my refusal to accept that I was medically ill and an anorexic had hampered our therapy. I was completely devastated that this was how the so-called Eating Disorder Specialist for my health authority felt. If she couldn't help me, then who could? I really was now on my own – I felt abandoned, rejected and discarded.

My weight from that moment began to plummet quite quickly and I was left just seeing my dietician, and very occasionally my GP. The problem was that every time I saw them I thought that if they didn't mention my weight loss then it wasn't noticeable and therefore I hadn't lost enough. The result was that I was spurred on to lose even more weight. I then made a promise to myself to start swimming twice a day and if I was to eat anything more than I intended, I would swim an extra mile to burn it off.

I always knew when I was winning in achieving my goal, because the more ill I felt, the more successful I was in losing weight. Therefore, if one day I didn't feel too ill I knew I had eaten too much the day before. By the end of June all those days of feeling ill had paid off because I had lost a few more kilos and was ecstatic. I was exercising more and more, eating virtually nothing and even though I constantly felt awful that didn't matter to me because I was losing weight.

Inevitably work was not going well and one day I overheard two of the cleaners discussing with each other what a burden I was on Tony. Once again I thought everyone was against me.

My early mornings of starting at 5am to go swimming were almost killing me (and I'm not exaggerating). Frequently I would drive to the pool and sit in my car in the car park, trying desperately to get enough energy to walk the 50 metres or so from the car to the pool. Amazingly, though, I had the energy to swim mile after mile up to three times a day on top of a day at work. Sometimes the chest pains I experienced while swimming were really bad and I'm now convinced I was on the brink of having a heart attack. I was pushing myself to swim more and more, eating only fruit each day. By the time the summer holidays arrived I had swum 100 days in a row without a day off and was getting awards from the health and fitness club for being their most regular client. I now feel quite annoyed that a health and fitness club (of all places!) did not realise how abnormal it was for a person to swim three times a day, especially when so underweight. It should have been obvious I was obsessed with exercise and how ill it was making me.

No one in the medical profession had asked what my weight was for two-and-a-half months and during this time I had lost a lot more kilos. I was always allowed to tell the medics what my weight was, rather than have them weigh me, and if they didn't ask I didn't tell them.

My 29th birthday approached and during the week before I was constantly planning what I was going to eat to treat myself. I was determined that I wasn't going to lose control and eat more than I wanted, but it ended up all going terribly wrong. I did indeed eat more than I was happy with and was so angry with myself that for the first time I contemplated taking loads of laxatives. I had just experienced my first binge and my weight had gone up substantially in that one day. I was distraught with what I had done. I hated myself for being so weak-willed and was determined it would never happen again. If it did, I made up my mind I would just compensate with taking masses of laxatives.

In the middle of August 1997, I dislocated and broke my toe by hitting it on the edge of the bed. Mum and Dad had been due to visit for the day, so they took me to A&E where I was told I wouldn't be able to exercise for four weeks because of the injury. My whole world ended, I was devasted that I could no longer continue with my swimming and aerobics. I ended up having a row with my Mum in A&E because she just couldn't understand why not being able to exercise mattered so much to me. She told me that I was totally over-reacting and because of her obvious lack of understanding I ended up swearing at her; something I had never done before. She was stunned because this was so out of character for me: she ran out of the hospital crying. It was just two days before I started to swim again.

Towards the end of August I was severely underweight and was due to return to work in ten days as the summer holiday was coming to an end. I spoke to my dietician about my fears of returning to work, feeling as physically ill as I did. She told me that I had three options. First, I could stay the weight I was and get time off work again for being sick. Second, I could put on weight, put the anorexia behind me and return to a normal life. Or third, I could go into hospital. This was a shock to me as it was the first time that hospital had ever been mentioned. Deep down I knew I couldn't get out of this hole on my own, but for me the decision was whether I should continue to lose weight or fight it by getting help from a hospital. The dietician made an appointment for me to see a psychiatrist at the local adult mental health clinic, but it happened to be the same day I was due to start back at work. The hospital mentioned was an NHS hospital known as Clifftop Hospital, further along the coast, which had an eating disorder unit.

Sleep was becoming increasingly difficult due to my weight because I was always cold and couldn't get comfortable. The same was the case with having a bath. Even going to the toilet was hard because I would sit down on the loo seat and struggle to find the energy to stand up again.

It was around this time I received the letter from Tony that I have reproduced at the beginning of this book. Receiving it was really emotional. For the first time I got a glimmer of how my eating disorder was affecting other people. However, I was so caught up in my own world that I soon forgot about how upset he was and just carried on with the diet and exercise.

Just before seeing the psychiatrist at the beginning of September, I went to see my GP to get a sick note for work. She was shocked at how much weight I had lost since she last saw me. Unfortunately, this only spurred me on to thinking that I was doing the right thing in losing weight.

My depression was deepening and I was conscious of the fact that I couldn't keep this way of life up for much longer. I felt that hospital was my last ray of hope but was petrified that they would make me put on loads of weight and then discharge me feeling exactly the same way as I had before, if not a lot worse.

On 3 September 1997 I saw the psychiatrist that I had seen 18 months before. He made it clear to me that I had classic anorexia. He said he would write to the doctor at Clifftop Hospital in order for me to be admitted there. I took the opportunity to tell the psychiatrist my fears of being admitted - putting on weight, only to feel just as bad - if not worse - afterwards. He reassured me that at a higher weight I would not feel as bad. This later proved to be completely wrong.

The day after having this appointment with the psychiatrist I was livid with Tony. I found out that he had been to see my Mum and Dad without me knowing. He had decided that my illness was caused by them never telling me that they loved me. I was so angry and felt that I would never be able to forgive him or trust him again. He may well have been right, but I didn't feel it was his place to tell my Mum and Dad and upset them. The following day both Mum and Dad turned up at my house and told me that I had to believe them when they said they loved me very much but did not find it easy to say. I felt gutted that it had taken them 29 years to tell me that. I couldn't help also thinking that they had only told me because Tony coerced them into it and because they were convinced I was going to die. We all cried a lot that day, so it did at least help clear the air.

By the middle of September my weight had dropped even further and a new phase of my eating disorder began. I began to binge every two or three days, which caused me utter despair. I couldn't understand how I was losing all the control I used to have. I was left feeling even more repulsed by myself than before. The only way I could keep my weight low with the binges was by exercising more and with constant laxative abuse. I would take a huge amount of laxatives following a binge and that cycle of bingeing and then purging continued until I was eventually admitted into hospital in November. I found it very difficult admitting to the binge episodes. I was so appalled with myself that I had allowed it to happen and the thought of anyone else knowing filled me with panic.

The hospital admission was still being discussed, but after waiting months, a bed had still not become available: eventually my psychiatrist started looking into alternative hospitals.

I was sick of family members going behind my back. My brother and Dad were both ringing my GP and psychiatrist to find out why there was a delay in me being admitted. I was sick of a lot of things - sick of the treatment I wasn't getting, sick of my illness, sick of being 'fat and vile looking' and sick of people telephoning me. I wanted just to be left on my own; I had become a recluse in my home.

I started making up mantras that I would say over and over in my head all day long. These encouraged me in my weight loss attempts for a few days, but would inevitably end in a binge followed by two days on the toilet after taking vast quantities of laxatives. This cycle continued for the next two months.

On 1 October I had lost even more weight and my psychiatrist told me I finally had approval from the NHS to be funded for inpatient care, at a different hospital than was previously discussed. It was a private hospital called Forest Field. He asked me whether I still believed I wasn't anorexic. After leaving this appointment I remember thinking how clever I was in conning even him that I was indeed anorexic. In reality it was the anorexia conning me. Even though I had approval to be admitted to hospital, it was still some time before it happened.

I was feeling really ill all the time now and I frequently had bouts of what I can only describe as 'out of body experiences'. I also had an overwhelming fear that I would be admitted to hospital only to be discovered to be a fraud. I struggled to accept how I could be anorexic, eating the way I was as well as being as fat as I was. I was still swimming frequently and it was then that I began to notice that the hair on my head was falling out but that other parts of my body were becoming hairier.

My days continued to be spent planning when and how to exercise and what and when to eat; I could think of nothing else. I used to plan my binges down to what food I would buy, when I would buy it and where. Every morning I would wake saying the same mantra: "Today I am going to win – I am not going to let the 'bad' part of me get the better of the 'good' part." The 'bad' I considered to be eating, and the 'good' was starving myself.

The binge episodes were freaking me out. I was always debating with myself how much more I could take and whether I should kill myself. Nothing would be as bad for me as the total humiliation of going into hospital and being laughed at for being too fat.

One strategy I used to avoid these binges was to go out of the house every time I felt hungry. Walking was difficult – my legs were always shaky and I found it really hard to focus. I always thought I was going to collapse, but I just kept thinking of the calories I could burn up compared to just sitting in a chair. However, my bingeing was becoming such a regular occurrence that I couldn't seem to do anything to avoid it. One of my diary entries at the time sums up what my days consisted of:

'I've now spent the last three days in my bedroom – alternating between bingeing and then feeling sick and faint through eating too much, feeling totally depressed, crying, looking at myself in the mirror, thinking what a fat disgusting cow I am, running between my bed and the loo (because of the laxatives) and finally feeling totally desperate and distressed about the way I've been behaving.'

I found myself thinking more and more about ending it all. I just couldn't cope with how I felt after bingeing.

I had put on one kilo since the last time I had seen my dietician and because I felt so ashamed that I just couldn't face seeing her. I had to lose weight fast and the only way I knew how was to take more laxatives. One day when I was out buying the laxatives I experienced a panic attack. The tablets I had always bought were out of stock as they were being repackaged and no matter which shop I went to, they were unavailable. I was distraught as I knew that particular brand worked for me to lose weight. Eventually I had no choice but to settle for another brand: not surprisingly it worked just as well as my regular brand.

I eventually plucked up the courage to tell my dietician about my binges. She assured me that when you had anorexia it was very normal to do this. I had my doubts about that. My BMI was at a similar level to when other anorexics had died. I was told that my health was in real danger: both the dietician and my GP told me that the sooner I was admitted the better, as I desperately needed help.

I was eventually told by my psychiatrist that Forest Field Hospital would contact me in the next few days. I was panic-stricken: so many things were freaking me out. The list below sums up the thoughts going through my head at this time:

- I was too heavy to go in to hospital
- Other patients would laugh at me
- They would find out that I was a fraud
- I wasn't really anorexic
- I didn't want to be the fattest there
- They might turn me away at the hospital
- I didn't want to go
- How would I do my exercise?
- I wasn't thin enough to be anorexic
- What if my weighing scales had been wrong?
- The doctor would take one look at me and see that I wasn't underweight at all.

I got the phone call from Forest Field Hospital on 4 November 1997 and the following day Dad took me there to see the consultant psychiatrist who would be in charge of my care. I was nervous about meeting with him. First, he wanted to talk to me on my own and then with Dad present. He asked me hundreds of questions including my history of weight loss, whether psychiatric illness ran in my family (it didn't) and then personal questions about whether I made myself sick, whether I took laxatives, even whether I shoplifted or had a criminal record. The questions continued: about my sexual relationships, whether I heard voices, whether I had OCD or panic attacks, and then eventually my level of exercise. At the end of those endless questions the psychiatrist told me that there was absolutely no doubt that I was anorexic. I spoke to him about my concerns of putting on weight without 'my head getting sorted'. He said that he was unsure whether my anorexia was caused by the depression, or the depression was caused by the anorexia. He made it clear that I had to decide whether I wanted his help or not. I was then shown around the eating disorder unit and remember stupidly thinking that because each room had an ensuite bathroom I would be able to continue with my laxative abuse. I was even naïve enough to think I could 'escape' in the evenings to go running in the grounds without anyone noticing.

I had to wait until I had an admittance date. I continued to see my dietician who told me I was "such a lovely, intelligent girl" with such a future ahead of me, which was why I needed to take the help from Forest Field Hospital, even though no one could force me. This helped me make the decision to ring the psychiatrist from the hospital to say I was prepared to give it a try. He asked whether I was sure that was what I wanted and pointed out that there was no point in doing it only because other people wanted me to.

The next day I stocked up on laxatives, buying two packets at each chemist's I went to. My new mantra became: "Food is bad; food is evil; food is what makes me fat; food is what makes me detest the way I look." Ten days later I still hadn't heard from the hospital about a date to be admitted. I was feeling more and more desperate and began to think that the psychiatrist had changed his mind about helping me. Suicide was becoming the only viable option.

On 17 November my dietician rang to say the delay was because the NHS would only fund me for six weeks at the hospital, whereas the consultant psychiatrist wanted funding for thirteen weeks. The following day I got a phone call from him to tell me I was being admitted the next day. During that phone call I took the opportunity to tell him again that I was worried I was conning him. His reply was quite simply: "what do you mean – the fact you're seriously ill?" He said that he was no fool and I wasn't conning him in the slightest.

CHAPTER 5

A Time-Bomb Waiting to Go Off

Dad picked me up early in the afternoon on 19 November 1997 and we made our way to the hospital. I was nervous but also felt quite relieved that I was going to get help. There was a battle going on in my head as to whether I was doing the right thing or not and throughout the journey I was constantly seeking Dad's reassurance.

When I arrived, the Ward was really quiet because all the other eating disorder patients were in a group therapy session. That suited me – I didn't want to meet any of the others and end up comparing myself to them: I knew I would always feel bigger than they were. I had a few visits from the doctor and some nurses and was then told that my first meal would be dinner at 6pm. Dad left at that time and I was petrified.

My first dinner was awful; not only was I meeting the other seven patients in the unit for the first time, but over the last few years I had developed a phobia of eating in front of anyone else. Everyone ate in complete silence and the atmosphere was strained. It all got too much for me and at one point I walked out. I soon learnt that this kind of behaviour would not be tolerated and I was told that I would have to sit in the dining room for as long as it took me to finish everything on my plate (even if that took all night). As I hated any type of confrontation, I realised I had no alternative but to finish my meals.

After finishing my first meal, which took many hours, I went

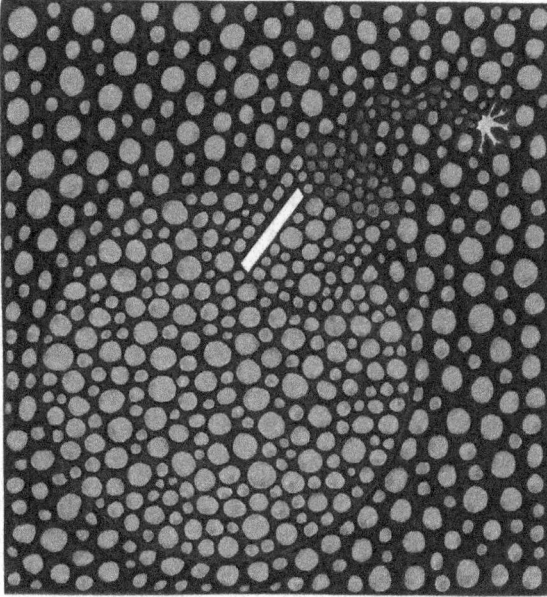

back to my bedroom feeling painfully full. I then discovered my bedroom window only opened four inches, so my plan to go running in the middle of the night was out of the question. I also discovered that my toilet door was locked. I had no idea how I would cope, not having access to a toilet in order to take my laxatives. Panic began to overwhelm me and to make matters even worse I was then weighed - for the first time during my whole illness - by someone else. I was told my weight in kilos but had no idea how that converted to stones and pounds. I hated the place already. One of the other patients was already getting on my nerves because she constantly complained about how much weight she had put on. I felt like thumping her because I was at least four times her size. I had only been at Forest Field for about five hours, but already it was all getting too much for me. I started to plan that I would walk out of the ward, then out of the front door of the hospital and go running in the grounds. I had to burn off all the food I had eaten at dinner and I stupidly thought that no one would even notice that I had gone. I was wrong about that – I soon discovered that there were CCTV cameras everywhere and I was very quickly escorted back to the unit and given a stern talking to.

The following morning we were all woken up at 7.15am, told to use the loo (which was unlocked for us) and then to line up in order to be weighed. I very quickly came to hate Mondays and Thursdays as they were the two days that we were weighed each week. The meal I had eaten the day before meant that my weight had gone up by 0.5kgs. I thought that at that rate I would be out of the hospital in a fortnight. After being weighed we had to go to breakfast and then attend the exercise class called 'Stretch and Tone.' I remember thinking that maybe things weren't all bad if we were allowed to exercise, but I soon learnt that what they called exercise and what I called it, were two completely different things. The exercises were very sedentary - I wondered what the point was because it would do nothing to burn any calories. So I decided that I would liven up my exercises by making them high-impact and as energetic as possible. I was very soon shouted at and told off for jumping and for not doing what I was told. I thought that was ridiculous and my anger towards the place escalated.

After the 'exercise' class we had to then go for 'snacks', which consisted of various quantities of biscuits dependant on the stage of recovery we were at. This was then soon followed by lunch (which to me was enormous). I then had to sit through my first group therapy session, which was called 'Diaries.' This lasted for two hours during which I was in agony because I felt so uncomfortably full from lunch. 'Diaries' took place three times a week and involved all the patients on the unit discussing with one another their feelings and fears and possible solutions to the problems they were experiencing. Although my first session was nerve-racking, I soon discovered that others felt the same as I did about food and their body image. I remember thinking that maybe I was anorexic after all. Some of the group members had, like me, been recently admitted, some had been at Forest Field for some time, while others were soon to be discharged. So inevitably among us there was a variety of body weights and shapes.

After 'Diaries' we all had to have 'snacks' again with yet more biscuits. Feeling very pleased with myself, I managed to hide a biscuit up my sleeve and fling it out of my bedroom window. However, I couldn't even do that successfully, as it was soon discovered by one of the nursing staff. We then had dinner which took me over two hours to finish. I couldn't handle the awful negative thoughts I was having, so straight after dinner I escaped the ward and hospital for another run. Once again, I was caught, but that didn't stop me trying again at 2am when I couldn't sleep. No matter how many attempts I made, I always got caught and escorted back to the ward.

That second day at Forest Field (my first full day) turned in to the worst day of my life. All the coping mechanisms I had to avoid food or get rid of it if I had eaten, had been taken away from me. I was unable to get away with anything. I wasn't sure that I could handle it and had serious second thoughts about what I had agreed to by coming to Forest Field Hospital.

The next day I had the biggest shock of all – I woke up and felt hungry. I couldn't understand how that could happen when I had eaten so much over the last couple of days and had felt so overly full. I was completely freaked out. I felt angry at what the hospital had done to me and I behaved in a constantly aggressive and hostile way. That day I had a visit from my consultant psychiatrist who told me in no uncertain terms that there were three options available to me – to discharge myself, to go home and to think about what I wanted (they would keep my bed for 48 hours), or to stay and start to play by the rules. I was being treated as a child but looking back I can see that was how I was behaving. I was also told I was banned from attending 'stretch and tone' because the teacher didn't like my attitude. I was fed up and hated everyone.

I ate my dinner more quickly that evening and was congratulated by the other patients because of it. I couldn't understand why I was being congratulated when I felt I should be punished for eating it. When I got back to my room I made myself sick and cried for the remainder of the evening.

I began to feel paranoid – not only was I incredibly fat, but I felt all the others disliked me. Mum and Dad were due to visit the following day and all I could think about was hoping that they wouldn't come because they would surely notice the amount of weight I had put on. I didn't want them to see me fatter. I imagined they would be as disgusted with my body as I was. My mind was in turmoil. I wanted to get better … as long as I didn't have to put on weight.

I was distraught the next day about Mum and Dad seeing me and was hysterical. The nurses had to give me some Valium to calm me down, which did help a lot. I was also worried about the 'weigh in' the next day. I had now been at Forest Field Hospital for four days and with all the food I had eaten and with no exercise and no laxatives, I was panic-stricken as to how much weight I had gained.

After a sleepless night, the 'weigh in' the next day showed that I had put on a massive 2.6kg. I was appalled and horrified. The nurse who weighed me told me that the aim was for me to put on 1-1.5kg a week. So how come I had put on 2.6kg in four days? I was angry with them, but more so with myself for allowing that to happen. I took out the laxatives that I had sneaked in when I first arrived – and took loads of them. The problem was that I had to tell the staff what I had done because of repeatedly needing my toilet unlocked. Initially the staff nurse on duty refused to unlock my toilet. I soon grew to dislike that woman and the next day her attitude was totally summed up when she said quite openly that "all anorexics are childish and attention seekers". I couldn't believe (and still can't) that a staff nurse working in an eating disorder unit would have such an attitude.

Having no control over my food intake was terrifying. There was nothing I could do to get the control back unless I left the hospital, but then I knew I would have no chance of recovery.

I was threatened with being discharged if I used laxatives again. By the end of November, I had my first 'weigh in' where I didn't put on any weight; in fact I had stayed the same as the previous time. I was totally elated, but this was very soon shattered when I was informed that because of my lack of weight gain, my portion sizes would increase so that I was on a total of 3,000 calories a day.

I continued to feel angry, ashamed, guilty, embarrassed, depressed, totally out of control and helpless. I had so many emotions going round my head all the time; so much so that I began to think I was going mad. When the staff congratulated me for finishing a meal, I used to say to myself "but it's not well done at all, is it? It would be well done if I hadn't eaten it."

Around that time, my consultant decided that I should start four new therapy groups during the day: coping with depression, assertion, psycho-drama and art therapy. I continued to argue with him about my portion sizes and he would continually say that even if I put on 2.5kgs at the next 'weigh in' he still wouldn't reduce my calorie intake.

On 1 December I had put on another 1.4kgs, which was a total of 3.6kgs in twelve days. I was angry, but worse than that, I was disgusted with myself. My anger continued when my consultant told me that my room was far too cold and unless I stopped opening the window, he would nail it shut. He even had a nurse put a thermometer in my room because he was sure I was purposely making the room cold so I would burn more calories by trying to stay warm. The thought hadn't even entered my head. Even when I told the truth I still wasn't believed and shortly after that warning, the window was indeed nailed shut.

My clothes were starting to feel tighter, which really scared me. It again reinforced just how weak-willed I was in allowing weight-gain to happen.

I was, however, beginning to gain a bit more confidence with the rest of the group and on one 'diary session' even told them about my chaotic eating habits prior to admission. The problem was that afterwards I experienced so many disturbing emotions – I felt exposed, vulnerable, ashamed, disgusted, vile, gluttonous, angry and worried sick what the others would think of my revelation. My mind was in turmoil and that evening I felt suicidal.

My original fears of going into hospital and gaining weight without my 'head being sorted' had now become a reality. I felt that the weight was going on too fast and because of that there was no time for my 'head' to be sorted. I'd hit rock bottom. The thoughts and feelings in my head were getting more negative and destructive by the day. However, the consultant did eventually agree that he would lower my calorie intake if I put on too much weight in the following day's 'weigh in'.

That day arrived and it was a complete disaster. I ended up putting on another 1.3kg. I was livid and stormed off to the nearest village (just down the road from the hospital) and bought boxes of laxatives from the chemist. I also bought painkillers. I couldn't cope any longer and ended up taking one whole packet of tablets thinking I would kill myself. But it was useless – I couldn't even do that right. I just ended up having to see the general doctor who told me I hadn't taken enough to cause myself any harm. She was not at all happy with me and made that very clear. A few hours later the staff nurse on duty came to see me and told me that I had to try and get the good voices in my head to be louder than the bad voices. Although I wasn't schizophrenic, I always had those two voices going on in my mind – one telling me what I should do and the other telling me what I shouldn't do. The consultant did, however, reduce my calorie intake after that and decided to put me on the drug fluoxetine, an anti-depressant.

Tony had been visiting twice weekly since I had been admitted to the hospital (usually one evening during the week and once at the weekend). One diary entry that I wrote on 6 December was: "half of me doesn't want him around me at all and then half of me is so scared of being without him … I don't know whether my feelings are due to the anorexia or whether they are 'real' thoughts … my thoughts seem as screwed up as my thoughts around anorexia". It became clear that I couldn't think straight or rationally about anything; thoughts went round and round my head continuously without a decision ever being made.

One day the consultant made me write a list of everything I avoided wearing. My list was endless. I was renowned for wearing everything big and baggy and never showing off any flesh. All the clothes I wore were black or dark navy. I also wrote that I never tucked shirts into my trousers; admitting this was a mistake because from then onwards the consultant nagged me to tuck them in, so as to confront my fear of my bum looking big in anything I wore. I refused.

Fear of the dreaded 'weigh in' never went away. I came to the conclusion that if I put on weight, I felt horrendous; if my weight stayed the same all I could think about was losing it; and if I lost weight (which was what I really wanted) the consultant would raise my calories again. It was a no-win situation.

On 8 December I did, for once, lose 0.5kg, but then the consultant didn't believe that the loss was natural. Even when I did stick to the rules no one ever believed me. He suggested that I think about staying in the hospital over the Christmas period (as I had previously told him my Christmas dinner the year before consisted of two peas and a five-hour walk).

By 11 December my weight meant that I had less than 6.5kg to go until I reached my target weight set by the hospital. At 5' 4" that was the lowest weight considered to be healthy. In three weeks I had put on 4.8kgs, which totally appalled me. I panicked when I realised that I could no longer use one hand to encircle the top of my arm, or get two hands around the top of my thigh!

I found it increasingly difficult to get dressed in the mornings. Even though there were no mirrors in the unit, I felt fat in everything. I couldn't face people seeing me that way. When I told my consultant how I felt, I was accused of "not talking intelligently".

Eventually I had my first decent conversation with the 'stretch and tone' teacher. She said that one thing she had observed was that weight gain was accompanied by a much less hostile attitude.

By the middle of December my weight gain had at last slowed down and meant that I had put on less than 0.5kgs in ten days. That was superb news for me, but not for my consultant who once again soon increased my calories.

After much deliberation, I decided to stay in hospital over Christmas. I thought it would be less stressful not only for me but also for my family, who I was sure were dreading me visiting.

On 17 December it snowed and I enjoyed a rare bit of excitement as a group of us had a snowball fight outside. However, all I could think about was that I wasn't making full use of my ten-minute walk (which I was now allowed twice a day.) I also felt guilty about smiling and laughing and having a good time – I felt that I didn't warrant it as I had allowed an awful negative thing to happen to my body (weight gain.)

Constant disagreements continued with the consultant about my calorie intake - I thought my calories should have been lowered, he thought they should stay the same or go up. Our sessions together began to focus on the future and whether I would come back, after discharge, to the hospital twice a week as a day-patient, or go back to seeing my old dietician and psychologist in the community. I told him that I was keener on being a day-patient, as I thought that in the long term that would help me more.

As my weight rose, I became more and more desperate. I would often ring Tony and ask him to take me home for the day (which I was allowed to do every now and again at that stage) with the sole purpose of being able to buy some laxatives. I was once again banned from 'stretch and tone' for "having the wrong attitude." I was overcome with panic and depression at how big I had allowed my legs to become and that hideous fact was all I could focus on. Apparently my behaviour was "detrimental to the rest of the group" and that was why I was banned from 'stretch and tone'.

As most of us were finding that our clothes were getting too tight, it was decided that we could have a trip out to the local Marks and Spencer. The problem was that, even before we arrived, I knew it was going to be a traumatic experience, as none of us had seen ourselves (with our new bigger bodies) in full-length mirrors. I certainly hadn't for a month, and then I had been one stone lighter. I knew I wouldn't cope well and that proved to be the case. Although it was nice to buy some new clothes, I just felt repulsed with how I looked in the mirrors and was devastated to buy a size bigger than I had been used to. I couldn't get that out of my head and it haunted me for weeks afterwards.

My constant urge to escape and buy laxatives was overwhelming. The day after clothes shopping, I walked into the village to buy some laxatives but to my dismay the shop was shut. I couldn't believe my bad luck, and what made it worse was that none of the staff at the hospital knew I had gone, so that certainly felt like a huge opportunity missed.

One of the nurses supervising us that day for our evening snacks was a rather large woman. While supervising us, she ate the same biscuits we were forced to eat. I just couldn't get out of my head why anyone would willingly eat them, let alone like them. I also convinced myself that by eating them, I would end up being as fat as her.

Every time Mum and Dad came to visit, I was convinced they would see me as getting fatter and more unattractive. In reality, they couldn't have been more pleased (and I'm sure relieved) with the way I was beginning to look.

I was again banned from 'stretch and tone'. It seemed that every time I was allowed back, I would once again be banned a couple of days later. I was yet again told that I jump, I'm aggressive and hostile "which is detrimental to the rest of the group." My mood continued to get worse by the day. I was beginning to feel that there was no light at the end of the tunnel … and things were just getting harder and harder.

I was told I had to speed up my eating because all I was doing was "prolonging the agony". My consultant asked me if it was all getting too much, and whether I wanted to quit the programme. Although that was very tempting for me to do, I still held on to the vague hope that maybe I could get better, even though at the time that seemed to be more and more of an impossibility.

On Christmas Day we were weighed: I had put on 1.8kg in a week and was now getting close to my target weight. My whole body felt bruised, but I was assured by the staff that this was normal during weight gain. All over Christmas I just couldn't get out of my mind that I had put on 7.3kg's in five-and-a-half weeks. I felt at breaking point. To make it worse, I began to feel hungry after my evening meal: this was terrifying and fears of not being able to stop eating entered my head.

Yet again, at the end of December I told my consultant my fears that I was putting on all this weight but that my 'head state' was worse, not better, than before I was admitted. He admitted that it was worrying him too, and that he was prepared for me to stay beyond the time it took to reach my target weight. At the end of the day, funding was the main issue. I had lost 0.7kg at the 'weigh in' that day, so (surprise, surprise) my calories were increased yet again. He asked me to write a list of all the advantages and disadvantages of anorexia that I could think of. My list of advantages still outweighed (pardon the pun) the disadvantages. To me, anorexia still seemed a very attractive option.

I had a nice surprise visit from my dietician a few days after that and she told me that my consultant was extremely worried about my "appalling distorted body image". If he'd said that to her, it proved to me that he didn't know how to cure me - and that was scary.

I was told that if I was still wanting to lose weight, then I was wasting my time being in hospital. I felt that the consultant was implying that he was going to abandon me as he had run out of ideas of how to treat me. I was left wondering whether there was anyone who could help me.

I had a visit from Tony that evening. I allowed him for once to hug me, as long as he didn't put his arms around my waist or bum. Those were the areas of my body that I thought were the most fat and I couldn't run the risk of him feeling it. Once again I was worried he would be repulsed by my fat. That hug was a major step forward, though, as I hadn't allowed him to touch me for a very long time.

Discussions were going on as to where I was going to live when I finally left the hospital. My consultant didn't think it would be a good idea for me to stay with my Mum and Dad (which I agreed with) so it was discussed whether I lived with Tony or my brother (who lived in the Midlands). I wanted to live on my own – I was an adult and I had my own house, after all. I think he thought that I would never cope on my own, but all I wanted was to be left alone with no grief from anyone, so I could lose weight again (which was obviously what he was trying to avoid).

I was extremely close to my brother when we were in our twenties and knew that he was very concerned I was anorexic. I could speak to him about anything and that continued until 2003 when he had children and his life began to centre on them. Living a long distance apart also meant that we saw each other a lot less. However, at the beginning of 1998 he came to visit me in the hospital: I very much looked forward to seeing him. He took me out for the day and we went shopping. Once again, I was able to find the opportunity to secretly buy laxatives and sneak them back into the hospital.

The following day I lost 0.5kgs, which meant that my calories were raised. I was livid with my consultant yet again. In 'Diaries' that afternoon, I read out my Step 3 (we followed the '12 steps to success' programme during our inpatient stay, which Alcoholics Anonymous also used at that time). This consisted of writing approximately twenty sides of A4 charting how my illness had affected my life and that of others close to me. My consultant read it immediately afterwards. He did later comment that it gave him "a greater insight into how desperate things had become" for me.

My mood got a lot worse on 8 January when my weight went up a massive 1.9kg from the previous 'weigh in' of three days before. I couldn't stop crying and felt so desperate. I was 2.3kgs from my target weight and my head was in a worse state than it had ever been before. I was intent on discharging myself and was inconsolable. Even my consultant couldn't understand the weight gain and agreed that I should be weighed again the next day (which was unheard of). The following morning it had dropped by 0.7kg, so at least I felt a bit happier about that.

During those difficult times I wrote in my diary that "somehow recovery doesn't seem an attractive option anymore – in fact reverting back to anorexia seems much more attractive."

In eight weeks I had put on a total of 8kgs. I felt that my consultant had given up on me because when I spoke to him about how I felt, he didn't respond. Instead he told me that he wanted me to start going swimming with the 'stretch and tone' teacher. There was no way I could contemplate doing that because of the way I felt about my huge body and I couldn't believe that he would even suggest it.

I was then told that I had funding to stay as an inpatient until the middle of February.

On 17 January, Tony took me out for the day. He told me that it wasn't until he thought he was going to lose me that he realised he loved me. I thought that was such a lovely thing to say even though I couldn't understand how anyone could possibly love me, given the size I had become.

Eating while on 'leave' was difficult. I found that the guilt of eating in hospital was reduced considerably because it was out of my control, but as soon as the choice of how many calories I ate was given back to me (and I was in control) all those feelings of guilt came flooding back.

Mum and Dad visited me on the 26th. The first thing Mum said to me was "what have you done to your hair? It looks really flat."

To me, this just summed up her complete insensitivity. I couldn't understand why, knowing how self-conscious I was, she would ever say that (even if she may have thought it). She just spoke her mind time and time again with no appreciation of how it made me feel.

As soon as my weight didn't go up on 'weigh ins', my calories were increased, my toilet was once again locked, and walks were restricted or stopped completely. My fluoxetine was upped to the maximum dose and I was put on a drug that is no longer prescribed, called thioridazine. This drug was prescribed mainly to schizophrenics as it treated disturbed and unusual thinking, loss of interest in life and inappropriate emotions.

In one session with my consultant I was asked if I ever wore skirts. I told him that I used to, because Tony liked it. His response was: "Was that because he wanted to see your ugly fat legs and for everyone else to laugh at them?" I'm sure that he wanted me to realise how stupid I was being, but I felt that he was taking the mickey out of me by being sarcastic. The hate I sometimes felt towards him became worse when he told me that he wanted me to start eating in the main dining room of the hospital, with all the other patients and staff, not in the eating disorder dining room where I had been eating up to that point. I couldn't believe how insensitive that was, when he knew I had a phobia of eating in front of other people. Now, of course, I realise that was exactly why he wanted me to do it. I did think that I might get away without eating so much food in the dining room, but very soon learnt that the canteen staff were monitoring me and reporting back to my consultant.

On 5 February 1998 I not only reached my target weight but went over it by 1.1kg. I was revolted, disgusted and confused. That morning I walked out of the hospital and contemplated running in front of a car or lorry passing on the busy road at the end of the drive. I just wanted this hellish life to be over. I desperately wanted help … but no one could help me. That day I drew a picture of my gravestone and was overwhelmed by thoughts of killing myself.

I was told by my consultant that he was going to apply for further funding for me. My anti-depressant was changed as he now thought I had general depression as well as depression from the anorexia. I became anxious about the funding situation and the fact that it was all down to money whether I stayed or left the hospital.

By the 19 February my period had re-started and that depressed me even further. I had been dreading that day for the last two years, as it now proved I was a normal and healthy weight.

By the beginning of March my weight had gone 1.5kgs over my target. I was now eating all three meals a day in the main dining room of the hospital: I was furious with my consultant for continuing to make me do that and was often rude to him. I finally heard that I had funding to stay until 20 March and hence that day was set as my discharge date.

For the first time my consultant saw some of my artwork. At that time, the only way I was able to cope with my destructive thoughts and feelings was to draw what was going on in my head: it was something I continued doing for the following three years. Other people had told me that the drawings were very expressive in illustrating how I was feeling, but the comment I got from the consultant was that I was just reinforcing my poor body image. Was there anything I did that he agreed with? He told me I should stop the drawings and focus on more positive things.

Since my weight was way over target, I was put on a reduced food intake of 1,750 calories. My consultant told me that he knew how bad I was feeling but I did not believe that he did. He hadn't helped me to sort out my mental anguish and I had the feeling that he had given up on me. All he had done was to pile on the weight. Once again, I felt let down by the medical profession. He was supposed to be one of the top eating disorder specialists in the country and I felt that if he couldn't help me, then no one could. Despite what he had said about my drawings I decided to continue with them as I found them therapeutic.

I was getting nervous about my discharge, but also looking

forward to it, as I had no intention of staying at my target weight. I now knew that 'my head' was not going to get sorted. The consultant continued to tell me off for things I said or did and complained constantly that I walked "like an angry anorexic". In reality, that was exactly what I was. I now felt worse and more desperate than I had before being admitted.

On 20 March 1998 I left Forest Field Hospital as an inpatient and became a day-patient, attending two days a week. During those days I would have to arrive at the hospital by 10am, immediately be weighed, and then eat the same food the inpatients had to eat on the unit. I would have to attend the 'Diaries' session in the afternoon and have a consultation with the psychiatrist. I was then allowed to go back home after the evening meal (usually about 7pm). I hated attending as a day-patient because two days of eating all that food interfered with my diet schedule and although I got a buzz from losing weight on the 'weigh ins', it usually ended with a stern telling off and threats of being discharged. I didn't really care at that point if that happened to me, as my mind was again in turmoil and I could no longer deal with the negative thoughts I was having about my size.

I did, however, continue to attend day hospital until the end of July 1998 but my heart just wasn't in it. I continued to lose weight (albeit slowly) and possessed no set eating pattern during the days I wasn't at the hospital. I became addicted to 'pick and mix' sweets and survived just on those with no other real food. I found that my weight didn't go up if I ate sweets instead of food but this addiction to sweets soon caught up with me as I ended up having to have constant fillings at the dentist. On one occasion, I was told that I had eleven holes in my teeth. This was a complete nightmare as I had a huge fear of the dentist! Eventually I had to have nearly all my top teeth crowned and bridged, as well as having quite a few extracted because they were so rotten.

My weight dropped again in June. I was once again bingeing and felt that I was in a living hell all day every day. My depression was awful and most of the time I could only ever see one way out – that was to kill myself so that then, at least I would be able to get a release from the awful thoughts I was having.

By the middle of July, I began to miss my appointments at day hospital. The first time I couldn't face being weighed because I knew I had put on 1kg. I was so ashamed and couldn't bear the thought of anyone else knowing. My brain was overloaded with bad thoughts and it was around that time that I began to contemplate self -harming – I needed to punish myself for being so weak around food. I kept getting an overwhelming urge to cut my legs and arms, to try and cut all the fat off my body. The next time I was due to go to day-hospital, I couldn't face it. The next thing I knew, my GP came and knocked on my door as the hospital had contacted her. I didn't answer the door because when I felt that bad I would never answer the door or telephone, but would shut myself away from the outside world. The GP left a note and asked me to contact the surgery. I remember thinking how nice she was but even though that was the case, she still couldn't help me feel better.

My last day as a day-patient was on 27 July 1998. The consultant said to me that day: "I expect you are angry with me for not curing you." Yes, I was angry and felt that I was in a much worse place than I had been back in November when I was admitted: I had all the same thoughts but now had a much heavier body, which repulsed me. It was horrible saying goodbye to everyone, though, because I had made some good friends over the last nine months. Once again, I felt totally on my own in battling the anorexia and depression.

CHAPTER 6

The Unsupportive Support Group

B y now I had handed in my resignation at work. I had been on sick leave for a year: six months on full pay followed by six months on half pay. I knew that I wasn't well enough to go back to work in the September and I didn't want to take advantage by going back for one day and therefore being entitled to another six months off. So I decided that it would be better for me to resign. That should have been a really big deal in my life, but I was so obsessed with losing weight that it didn't even get a mention in my diary. I had a one-track mind that only ever included one thing – the quest to be thinner. I had started to claim sickness benefits when I left Forest Field Hospital and this became my only source of income.

In August my weight had gone up to 1.5kgs over what was my target weight while in hospital. That was terrifying because Tony and I were about to go to Spain on holiday and I had no idea how I was going to cope with wearing a bikini and eating out in restaurants every night.

I was once again seeing my dietician on a regular basis but when I couldn't face her because I'd put on weight, I simply would not turn up. That began to happen more and more often. I had always been such a reliable person, but since having anorexia, if I couldn't face someone or something, I would run away from it. This running away happened a lot if Tony wanted us to go to a social function –

more often than not I would make sure I wasn't at home when he came to pick me up. I had developed a social phobia and very rarely could I face seeing anyone. I was always worried what other people would think of the way I looked and therefore just avoided the situation.

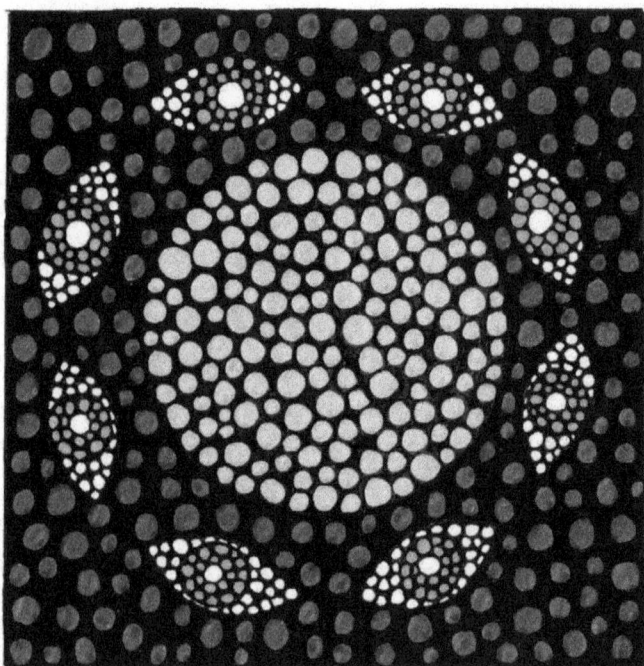

I feel everyone is staring at my fat,
disgusting and repulsive body

During that time my self-hate got worse and worse. My weight wasn't going down and the question I kept asking myself was: "Why do I no longer have the control and willpower I used to have to refrain from food, when I hate what I see even more than I used to?" I felt so out of control – I desperately wanted to lose weight but couldn't stop eating. The food was all tasting so good and fears of obesity plagued me. I was concerned that I wouldn't be able to stop eating and hence would get bigger and bigger. Before going into hospital that had been a big fear of mine and I now felt that it was becoming a reality.

On 14 August Tony and I went to Spain for our week's holiday. It turned out to be a difficult time for me. In my diary I wrote: "I should be happy I'm on holiday – but I just can't leave the anorexia behind". What I ate and what I looked like completely took over my mind. I thought what a terrible shame it was that I couldn't take a week's holiday from all my negative thoughts. I did, however, have my first alcoholic drink in two years, so I suppose I was acting like a normal human being in some respects. One day during that week Tony went off to play golf, so it meant I was on my own for most of that day. I questioned myself constantly about him leaving me that day and wondered whether it was because I was too fat and was embarrassing him. Or was it just because I was so boring and uninteresting that he would rather do something else? Those thoughts were typical of what went through my head every minute of every day.

One thing that shocked me during our holiday was that my sex drive returned. It was the first time in a couple of years that I could bear Tony to touch me and be intimate with me. However, Tony told me that he now didn't want to have sex before marriage because - a few years before - he had become a Christian. I blamed myself for that: I thought I had left a 'hole' in his life because we did not have a normal boyfriend–girlfriend relationship. I thought this 'hole' in his life had to be filled with something and that something became religion. We spent some time talking about The Alpha Course, which he wanted me to do. I didn't really mind the fact that he had become a Christian, but I did find it annoying when he told me that others were praying for me. I used to think "yeah, right … like that's going to get me better."

In September of that year I went to stay with my sister, along with Mum and Dad, in Wales. My sister had a three-year-old daughter and I remember during our stay that my Mum kept saying to my niece that she really loved her. I just wanted to shout out: "Why the hell didn't you ever say that to me?" It made me angry - after all, if she could say it to my niece then there was only one reason why she could never say it to me and that was because she didn't love me. One good thing about my time in Wales was that my sister had recently adopted a golden retriever called Bella. She had been re-homed numerous times because she would run off and chase sheep. The local farmers had threatened to shoot her, which was the reason why my sister had taken her on. However, she had her hands full with work and with bringing up a young child, so I began to think about offering Bella a good home. I was supposed to be staying with my sister for a fortnight, but after a week it all started to get too much for me. In my diary I wrote: 'When I feel like this I just want to be on my own with no hassles – to hide from the outside world and all its complications and difficulties.' In the end I asked if I could be taken home. I had already planned that I would start a new diet as soon as I got back.

Once I got home from Wales, I started to worry about a new therapy group I was going to be attending – it was a group for anorexics that was run by my dietician and the psychologist who I saw before I went into hospital. It was supposed to be a support group but I knew it would become an 'unsupportive group' for me, as I would feel the biggest person there and be self-conscious.

My depression had become bad again. I quite often would spend time on a nearby motorway bridge trying to pluck up the courage to end it all by jumping into the oncoming traffic. At this time it was agreed I would have Bella and so I drove to Bournemouth to pick her up from where my sister was staying on holiday. I thought that this could help my depression and give me a new focus in life.

A short time later I decided to stop taking my anti-depressants. I was finding it hard to lose weight at that time and thought that, as one of the side effects of taking the tablets was weight gain, it was best to come off them.

At the end of September I had lost 2kgs in a week. Things were looking up.

In the October I decided to visit two friends I had met in hospital. One had been re-admitted to Forest Field and the other – Emily - was in a general hospital being fed through a tube into her stomach. After visiting both friends, I knew that I didn't want to go back to hospital, but I did feel envious of the obvious control they both had in order to lose much more weight than I could.

Thoughts kept entering my head that if only I could lose just over 6kgs everything would be OK – I was absolutely sure I would be happier and less concerned at how awful I looked all the time.

At the end of that month I went back to Forest Field again, to visit the friend who had by now been transferred back from the general hospital. I was in shock after seeing Emily; at such a low weight she had totally lost her mind and made no sense when I talked with her. It was the first time I had experienced that happening to an anorexic. I was convinced she was about to die. Even though I was really shaken up, the experience still did nothing to stop my quest for weight loss. My thought was that there was no way I would ever get to the same state that Emily was in, therefore there was no similarity to my situation.

Tony was cross with me because I had not stuck with the Alpha Course that he had persuaded me to start. I just had no room in my head for anything other than losing weight. Tony was convinced that the Alpha Course was my only way out of anorexia, but I thought he was in cloud cuckoo land and that he was the one who was deluded, not me.

By November my depression was once again a real problem. The entry in my diary summed it up quite well: 'Life is such a struggle most of the time, I just don't see the point in continuing ….the dark hole I'm in just seems to get bigger everyday'. I would spend all my day contemplating and planning ways to kill myself - I saw no other option. I felt angry a lot of the time. My consultant at

Forest Field Hospital would often say to me "How sad it is that you are so angry with the world and everything that goes on in it."

On 20 November I decided to start a hunger strike. All my thoughts at that time focussed on the fact that the year before, I was 13kgs lighter. For the next few days I started eating very few calories a day and soon became the lightest I had been since the previous July.

By December I was feeling really unwell. I was once again feeling cold all the time; my eyes began to struggle to focus and I felt panicky, faint, and extremely tired. I felt so ill. I just wanted to be looked after, but I had no one to do this - I felt so alone with my struggles. I constantly pushed Tony away as I felt he didn't understand the thoughts I was having.

One day when I went to the support group, I walked out halfway through. The psychologist had really upset me by talking about my weight in front of the other anorexics. She made the revulsion I felt towards myself ten times worse. I was so confused – half of me wanted to be just left on my own, the other half wanted to get out of this hell-hole. I asked the same question to myself over and over again: "Why can't life be kind to me for once rather than always getting me down?"

I began to isolate myself more and more and decided to spend Christmas Day on my own. That way I thought I could carry on with my diet, without the worry of possible family arguments.

On 27 December I decided to make a New Year resolution that 1999 was going to be a successful year for me in terms of weight loss. I'd lost count of how many times I had promised myself that I would start a new diet, or a hunger strike, or an exercise routine, but nothing I did was ever successful enough. I always let myself down by either eating too much or not exercising enough.

My drawings continued to be therapeutic and by the start of 1999 they began to take on a different style to that which I had done before. I had become obsessed with fat globules contaminating my body. My diary entry for that time stated: 'I'm sure my skin is going to rupture very soon and all the globules of fat will ooze out.' Because of that obsession, my drawings consisted of 'fat globules' creating an image of what I was thinking.

I described my life at that time as one of imprisonment and I couldn't understand why I had to live that way when others did not. I wrote in my diary: 'I feel God has it in for me ... what have I done in my life that has been so bad to be punished this way?' I felt that no one could feel as desperate and distraught as I did, unless perhaps they were being tortured, which is exactly what I felt I was going through.

My anxieties about attending the eating disorder support group continued. For me, each meeting was yet another time of total humiliation, sitting next to the others who are so skinny, just looking at them with envy and jealousy. I wrote about sitting next to 'other anorexics for whom, because of their control and willpower, I have nothing but admiration'. I think having those feelings was why I found that group so 'unsupportive' – my head was just not in the right place for me to benefit at all from the group.

By the end of January I started having regular panic attacks. Whenever I went out of the house, panic struck me, and every time when in a supermarket buying food, I would have a full-blown attack.

I was constantly trying to find ways in which I could adequately describe to other people how I was feeling. I was so unhappy and desperate but felt no one really understood me. I remember thinking that if someone just had a glimpse of how bad I felt, maybe, just maybe, they might be able to help me. My drawings did help people understand, but the problem was that not many people ever saw my artwork. I often described myself in my diary as a caged animal at a zoo, with the cage resembling my body – 'but an animal can be released (from the cage) but I can't – I'm stuck with it – living with it every second, every minute, every hour and every day'.

At the end of January I came to the conclusion that no one cared about my depression. I felt that everyone thought that because my body was a healthy weight everything was OK, but I had never felt worse than I did at that time.

In February I started seeing a new psychologist who I soon grew to like. I felt that he took me seriously (without ever taking the mickey) and he was really keen to see my drawings so that he could try to understand better how I felt. We quite often spoke about my parents and I remember him saying that until I break away from Mum and Dad and do exactly what I want to do, rather than what they think I should do, then this will continue to be a major problem for me. I was brought up to believe that Mum and Dad always knew best and to respect them at all times. The problem was, I don't think I ever changed from that viewpoint once I became an adult and I still thought that they knew best and that I should always do what they wanted me to do. Even years later - and now in my mid-50s - I still struggle with the issue of not always doing what I feel they want me to do.

Unfortunately, even though I really liked that psychologist, I only saw him for three months: I was so depressed at the time, which made communication really difficult, and our sessions became too unproductive for them to continue.

I soon realised that I was becoming agoraphobic. It seemed that every time I went out of the house, I thought I was going to black out, so in the end I just avoided going out. I also stopped answering the telephone as I felt that it invaded my privacy and it also took up too much energy to talk to other people. I often wondered why others couldn't just leave me alone.

Suicide was now a real threat. My diary entry regarding this was 'it's not that I want to die - I just want to stop the pain'. I felt that there was no other way.

By March I was still going to the support group meetings (albeit unwillingly). We were asked in one session to write a list of how bad we felt when we were panicky; which we then had to share with the rest of the group. As I read out my list, the psychologist who was running the group said "God, that's about as bad as it gets ...if you were being seen by a psychiatrist you would be on tranquilisers." I wondered if at last I was finally getting through about how bad I was feeling.

The next time I saw my dietician I cried for the whole session. I felt so depressed. She asked me whether I would consider being admitted to a General Psychiatric Hospital so that my eating could be normalised again. The hospital she was referring to had such an awful reputation that I point-blank refused. I felt there was no point in even considering it, because as soon as my weight increased then so too would my anxiety and depression. I remained very desperate and even contemplated stealing my Dad's thyroid tablets (which he was taking because of an underactive thyroid condition). I thought that this drug would increase my metabolism and so enable me to lose weight. Although I seriously considered it, I do remember questioning myself about how much lower I could get than stealing the drug that kept my Dad well.

I was constantly being told to go back on my anti-depressants, but felt that I couldn't risk it. I thought if I began to feel better in myself, I would be more likely to eat and hence put on weight. I longed to be able to have a decent conversation with Mum. I wrote in my diary: 'I want a Mum like other people have – someone you can talk to about anything rather than absolutely nothing'. Alas, it was never going to happen.

At the beginning of April, my dietician visited me at home and told me that she wanted me to see my old psychiatrist again (who I had last seen prior to going into Forest Field Hospital). Twelve days later I had an appointment with him. I told him in no uncertain terms that no one cared about my 'head situation' – they were only concerned if my weight dropped to a dangerous level, but that I had never felt so much at risk than I did at that moment. I also told him that I felt angry, let down, alone and that I was running out of the will to live.

My weight had actually dropped to the lowest it had been since the previous June. That evening I began self-harming. I planned my suicide and I wrote: 'I just wish I wasn't such a coward and could just get on and do it, instead of contemplating all the time – the longer I put it off, the longer I suffer, so really it is only me to blame for this prolonged pain'. I continually said to myself: "Just take the pills - don't complain about all this misery if you can't even take the easy step of swallowing some pills. Everyone has to go through things they don't want in order to make things better .. just do it, for God's sake."

My drawings were no longer working as a release from all my built-up frustrations. Self-harm was now all I was thinking about. I lost the will to want to communicate with anyone, except with myself by writing in my diaries. 'My mind has become obsessed with suicide,' I wrote. 'I feel at the point of a mental and physical breakdown.' Once again I began spending all day in my bedroom and stopped going to the support group. I was just tired of talking – I felt too emotionally exhausted to even try.

By the end of April I was missing lots of appointments. I wrote: 'I seem to have lost my nerve in seeing all the medical professionals. In the last two weeks I've missed two support groups, one appointment with my dietician and one with my psychologist. I just want to hide from the whole world, not just today but for good.' My mind was all over the place. For example I wrote: 'every thought seems to have negative consequences and the more I contemplate them, the more intense they all become, so because of that I just end up doing nothing.' I would spend all day with these thoughts going around and around in my head.

By the end of April, I came up with what I thought was the reason for my illness and also the reason for why my thinking was the way it was. I called it 'My Theory'. I thought I had at long last discovered the reason I was ill and was so sure that I had cracked the mystery that I proudly presented it to my psychiatrist when I saw him on 5 May 1999.

My Theory:

* I am depressed because it's my body's solution to preventing me from becoming obese. If I'm not sad I will eat, and so to try to stop this happening my head is protecting me
* If I go out of the house, I have panic attacks. This is my body's way of protecting the rest of society from seeing me
* If I am a bad person - ie defy the rules of going out or eating - my body punishes itself in the form of self-harm (so I suffer pain) or in feeling more depressed in order to prevent it happening again (or increasing the intensity of panic attacks to stress the point that I'm doing wrong)
* By committing suicide, my body is trying to eradicate me from society - for everyone else's good. Society would be better off with my extermination
* If I was to take antidepressants, it would muck up my mind and therefore these thoughts may diminish. But I can't allow that to happen because it wouldn't be for the good of everyone else. So, by resisting taking these drugs, I am doing the correct, moral thing and thinking about the rest of society.

After he heard my theory, he decided that I needed to go back into hospital. He told me that I seemed to be removing everything from my life which was preventing me from committing suicide. I think the final straw for him was when he heard that I was re-homing Bella, who I had only adopted the year before but had found her difficult to look after. He spoke about me being admitted to Forest Field again, but the thought of their routines and rules filled me with dread – if they didn't help me before, why should they help me this time?"

Tony's solution to my illness was always the same – to find God and ask for his help. My response was always the same. I thought surely if God exists, or is there, he already would have helped me. Why should I have to ask him? It wasn't until years later that I found the answer to that question and God became part of my life. I think if I'd had the room in my head for anything other than losing weight it would have helped me at the time to have had faith, but I had neither the 'space' in my head or the energy to even contemplate it.

When I was a teenager, there had been times when I'd explored Christianity. One Easter I'd gone on a retreat at a convent with my best friend who was a devout Catholic. I'd even attended the local Catholic Church for a time and felt at peace there. It wasn't long before I then started going to Sunday services at a C of E church close to where I lived. I was teased a bit by my brother and sister for going, but I ignored them and decided I wanted to get Confirmed. Unfortunately, soon after starting Confirmation classes, I joined the local hockey club on Sunday mornings and so did not go to church again until 2008.

When Bella was re-homed to an experienced owner by the Golden Retriever Rescue Society, four days after seeing the psychiatrist, it suddenly hit me that my life now had no purpose and no structure. I had nothing to keep going for. I was distraught saying goodbye to Bella. I felt I had completely let her down, like all her previous owners. I cried for days and never really forgave myself for abandoning her.

By the middle of May I was still waiting to hear about my second admission to hospital. I wrote in my diary: 'I'm just too exhausted to continue to live the life I am living. The way things are right now is making me feel like I'm dying inside.'

My sleep pattern was all over the place. I would sleep all day and be awake all night. I was tired at night but didn't want to go to sleep. Half of me felt I didn't deserve it because I'd done nothing all day; the other half of me really liked the peace and silence that I didn't get during the day. It was during one of those nights of being awake that I decided that if I didn't get funding to return to Forest Field Hospital I was just going to give up and admit defeat. Three days after that, I did see the consultant from the hospital. He told me I was chronically depressed - about as bad as it gets. One of the conditions he stated for me being re-admitted, was that I had to agree to go on any medication he decided was right for me. Later that day I got a phone call saying I was to be admitted the following day (19 May 1999).

CHAPTER 7

The Plan to Save my Life

As soon as I was re-admitted to Forest Field in May 1999, I was put on a variety of different drugs. I also had to agree to take sleeping pills at night, to prevent me from staying awake all night drawing. I fought against those sleeping pills and would often fall asleep at 1am or 2am with pen and paper still in my hands. At times, the side effects of the cocktail of drugs I was taking made me feel unwell but I wasn't allowed to change drugs until I'd given each one a try for two or three weeks. This was to see if the side effects would subside.

I held onto the hope that my second hospital admission would be different from the first and that I would get more help from the staff. I hoped that they would concentrate more on my depression than they had previously, because this time I wasn't at such a dangerously low weight. I was desperate not to end up in the same situation – that is, my head being in a worse state on discharge than on admission. So, although I was sceptical, while there was the slightest hope of help I felt I had to give it a try.

Due to my poor mental state, I didn't often write in my diary; instead, I totally immersed myself in my 'fat globule' drawings and would often complete three or four a day. For me the drawings were much less taxing than the writing.

My self-harm had got out of control. I was cutting my arms and hands every time I was disgusted with myself for eating. This was not an attention-seeking strategy, because very few ever saw any evidence of my self-harm. In my deluded mind, I thought that if I cut myself, the fat globules that contaminated 99% of my body would pour out. I also had the urge to punish my arms and hands because it was these, after all, that enabled me to put food in my mouth. It was as if the 'bad' person in me was constantly willing me to punish myself, because I deserved it. I found the cutting was a way to achieve a release of pent-up feelings of anger and disgust. Nothing else relieved me in the same way that self-harming did.

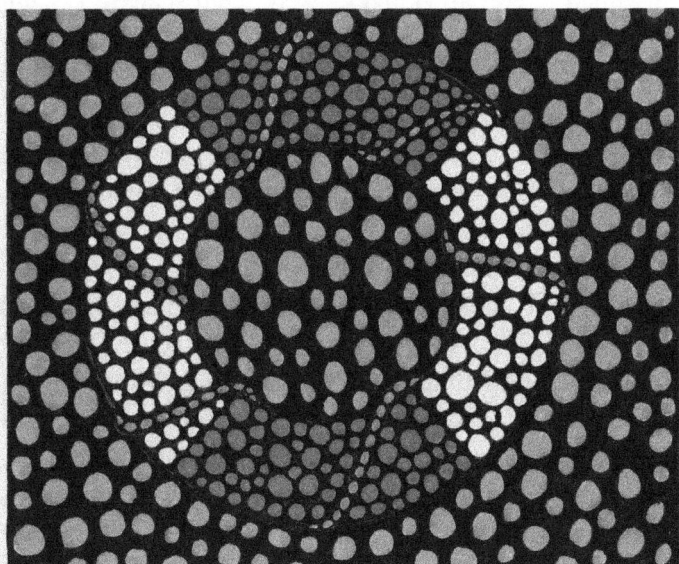

Will anyone be able to save me from drowning in anorexia and depression for the rest of my life?

I had only been at Forest Field Hospital for six weeks when I was told that my funding might stop. I couldn't believe it – it had happened again. I was at my target weight, but once again nothing had changed in my 'head'. Why was I ever so stupid as to believe that anything would be different this time? I felt that I had no other option but to commit suicide: I was just too exhausted to continue fighting anorexia any longer. So at the end of June 1999, I took a large overdose and ended up in the local general hospital for three days. When I realised that I hadn't been successful in my suicide attempt, I felt even more despair. I was sent back to Forest Field Hospital, but because of the funding situation I had no idea what the future held.

On 9 July I was caught red-handed self-harming. I was always so careful never to be caught, but my room was searched and my blades, which were art knives, were confiscated. I panicked– suddenly my comfort blanket and the only release that I had from the awful thoughts had been taken away from me. My consultant talked to me about ECT (electro convulsive therapy) and wanted me to think about having it. His reason was: "We are talking about saving your life." I didn't like the thought of having ECT, but I would have gone along with anything if it would stop my depression. However, when Tony found out what had been suggested, he put his foot down and was adamant that I was not going to have it. We had both loved the film 'One Flew Over the Cuckoo's Nest' and I think the scene in which McMurphy, played by Jack Nicholson, is forced to have ECT, haunted Tony. I was not in a sane enough position to go against him on that one.

At the end of July I began to walk in to the nearby village with staff to try to overcome my agoraphobia. That day another patient at the hospital had committed suicide on the main road by walking into the path of an oncoming lorry - as I had thought about doing on numerous occasions. I then began to believe that my thoughts caused harm to others and that became yet another thing I felt guilty about.

After I had been at Forest Field Hospital for three months, my consultant asked to meet with me and Tony together. At this meeting he told Tony that he had done all he could for me except give me ECT. Once again Tony refused to allow me to have it – instead he wanted me to speak to his vicar. I was not at all happy about this suggestion but somehow didn't have the energy to refuse. A few weeks later I met the the vicar and his wife, but felt extremely uncomfortable when they prayed for me: at that time, it was so out of my comfort zone.

On 19 August my diary entry read: 'I do get some glimpses where I feel I can beat this anorexia …but it's soon overpowered by the same old desperate thoughts.' Those glimpses completely vanished every time I put on weight.

I was due for discharge at the beginning of September and again my consultant wanted me to think about becoming a day patient, this time for five days a week not just the two that I had done before. I didn't want to do that and told him that I would come once a week to get weighed and to have a consultation with him. Over the next few days I conned my family and Tony by sounding positive about my recovery, when in fact I was looking forward to having the opportunity to lose weight again.

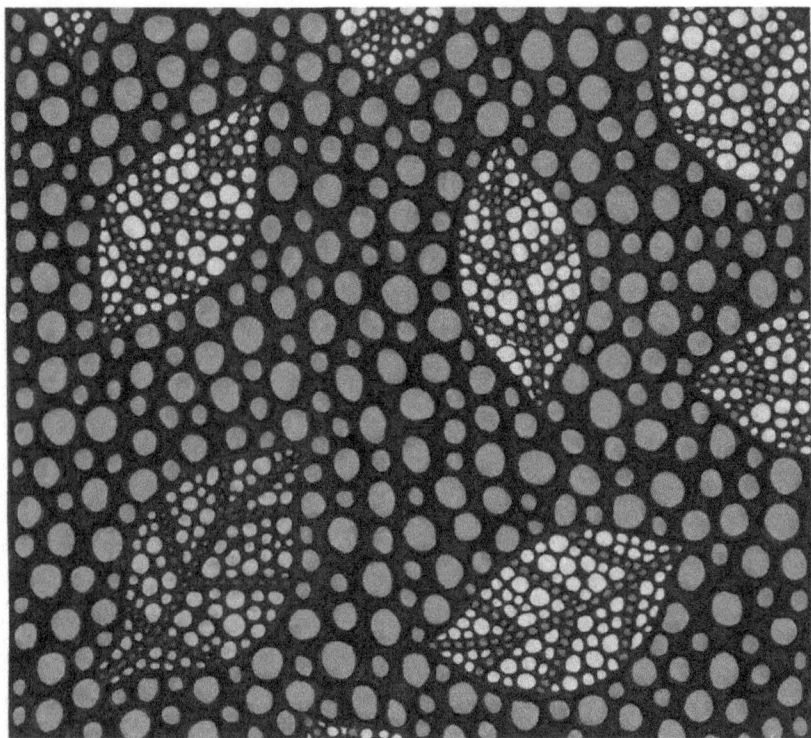

I feel like I am dying inside

CHAPTER 8
Unable to Cope

My first appointment with my consultant as an outpatient was on 6 September 1999. I also started to see my Community Psychiatric Nurse, who I had not seen for three years. She hadn't been able to help me back then, so I was doubtful anything would be different this time round. There were discussions about me re-joining the support group, but I was dreading it because I got so jealous of everyone (i.e. other anorexics) around me.

I was going to my local town centre every day for a latte. I was increasingly aware that this was becoming a ritual, even if I lived in fear of bumping into anyone I knew. I was worried what they would think of the weight I had gained since they had last seen me.

I was seeing my consultant on a weekly basis and he continued to be cross with me because I was losing weight (albeit only a small amount.) I decided that if I carried on seeing him, I had no option but to lie about my weight – otherwise he would refuse to see me. I hadn't binged for five months, but it still didn't stop me buying laxatives, just in case I needed them.

However, on 16 October, I did binge. I felt ashamed, embarrassed, angry, frustrated and despairing. I wanted to die. I stopped seeing my consultant at the end of that month because of lack of funding and that was the last time I ever saw him.

My mind continued to be in turmoil. My thinking was continually "I'm such a crap anorexic …things have got to change so I can become a success, not a failure." For me, success was losing weight and failure was gaining weight. My eating patterns continued to be hit and miss – typically I had a few days of starving, followed by an inevitable binge.

Tony and I were now seeing more of each other, but it still wasn't what I would call a 'normal relationship' – we rarely had any physical contact as I wouldn't allow it in case he felt my 'flabby bits'. For some reason Tony stuck with me, always believing that one day I would get better. At the time, I thought he was completely mad.

During the following six months it became clear to the medical profession that I wasn't coping and I was spoken to about being admitted to the local general psychiatric hospital called Warren Abbot Hospital. I was against it to begin with – I thought it would be full of 'nutters' (even though I had a psychiatric illness I still had an image in my mind of a typical psychiatric patient that was far from complimentary.) Although it is embarrassing to admit to that now, I think because I was always treated in an eating disorder unit rather than with general psychiatric patients, the stereotype was never challenged. I eventually agreed to be admitted, partly because I was so desperate to get help, but also because I hoped that as I wasn't going into a specific eating disorder unit, that would mean my depression would be the main focus for treatment rather than my weight. I also hoped that because it wasn't a specialist unit, I wouldn't feel the fattest there and wouldn't constantly compare myself to the other patients.

CHAPTER 9

Only Myself to Blame

For the next six months I was in a NHS-run general psychiatric hospital, very near to where I lived. Warren Abbot Hospital had 28 beds (male and female) and was therefore smaller than I had been used to. My consultant psychiatrist was the same one I had seen for the previous three years at the local adult mental health clinic when not a patient at Forest Field. During my stay at Warren Abbot I saw him weekly on the day he did his ward round. From the start, he told me that because the hospital was NHS run, I could stay as long as I needed in order to get better. That meant, straight away, the pressure was off to recover in a set number of weeks.

Initially I was scared about going to a general psychiatric ward. I had never mixed with patients who had schizophrenia, bipolar or personality disorders and I soon realised that some were very unstable. Before I was admitted, I imagined the hospital to be like the ones I had seen in TV documentaries. I soon found out that it wasn't nearly as bad as I had imagined.

On arrival I was shown to my bedroom, which is where I pretty much stayed for the next three days. It soon struck me that apart from seeing a doctor when I first arrived, no other nursing staff spoke to me. I remember thinking how different it was from Forest Field, where a nurse checked on me every 15 minutes - always going out of their way to make sure everything was OK and if I needed any support. Lining up for my drugs three times a day was the only time I left my room in those first few days, apart from to get a drink or to go to the loo – there were no en-suite rooms at this hospital. On the plus side it meant I didn't eat anything, as I chose not to go to the dining room at mealtimes. I thought if I could avoid doing that, the weight would drop off me. But on the third day of being there and, as I went to line up for my drugs at the nursing station, the staff nurse on duty erupted at me, saying that I'd eaten nothing since I'd been there and was making no effort at all. He told me that I might as well go home if I was not even going to try. He was right of course, but I thought at the time he showed no understanding. I was still desperate to get help but felt that could be achieved with me not eating – I didn't seem to appreciate that I couldn't get better from one without the other. After I had a stand-up row with the staff nurse in his office that evening, I agreed to make more of an effort.

The next morning, I went to the dining room with all the other patients. Eating with so many strangers was my worst nightmare – I just wanted to run away but couldn't bear having another row with the staff nurse, so I ate half a Weetabix and left. All those familiar guilt feelings as well as shame and disgust came flooding back in abundance, but in this hospital there was no one to support me through. I had no option but to immerse myself once again in my artwork to try to divert my destructive and dangerous thoughts.

Over the next week I ate most meals in the dining room (apart from skipping a few) but the portion sizes that I allowed myself were tiny. It soon dawned on me that it was a relief not to have to eat with other anorexics and I was stunned to realise how much 'normal' people ate. I had lost all sense of what a normal portion size was. For the last two years I had only ever eaten on my own or in hospital where I was on a weight-gain diet. Also, hardly anyone in Warren Abbot knew that I had an eating disorder, so I found it refreshing to eat with others that were unaware of this. All the competitiveness I was accustomed to, in eating with seven other anorexics, was now non-existent. Over time my appetite increased and I slowly ate more and more. I was still obsessed with not gaining weight, but without regular 'weigh ins' the stress was less intense. I was, however, still depressed and suicidal. I think one thing that made my depression so bad was that the only person I could now blame for my weight gain was myself – at Forest Field I always blamed my consultant because he was the one who controlled my calorie intake: now it was all down to me.

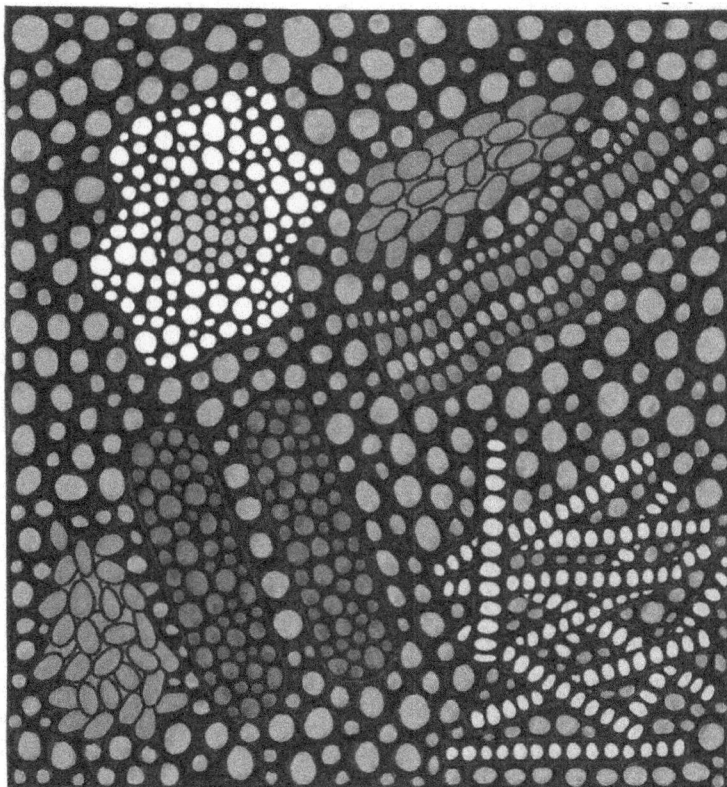

Why is a fry-up so appealing? The green represents my envy of the people who can eat it without putting on weight – or caring

Frequently, I would make a pact with myself that I would stop eating again so I could lose weight, but I seemed to lack the willpower and control I'd had in the past and was never able to sustain a starvation regime. At this hospital patients seemed to eat all the time, not just at mealtimes, so there was always food around, from which I could never escape.

I began to try and think of other ways I could lose weight. Some of the medication I was on at that time was renowned for causing weight gain, so I began to hide my medication, by not swallowing it and by spitting it out in the loo after I'd left the drugs room. After doing that for a week or so the nursing staff soon cottoned on and I wasn't allowed to leave the drugs room until I opened my mouth and proved to them that I had swallowed my drugs.

Not only was I eating more than I wanted to, I was also beginning to get a real taste for chocolate, which I had denied myself for so long. I began stockpiling it in my room – I would go out on 'leave' for a couple of hours with Tony and buy loads of chocolate from the nearest supermarket. Tony thought it was great because it proved to him that I was eating again, but I felt so out of control. Some nights I would eat three chocolate bars in a row: it all tasted so good and I just couldn't get enough of it. This lack of control made me hate myself and once again I began to feel that the only way out of all of it was to kill myself.

One night, I locked myself in the bathroom and took three boxes of a well-known painkiller (the only drug I had available). After doing that I went and sat outside in the communal garden, feeling distraught: I could not stop crying. Tony visited me that evening and kept asking me why I was so upset. Eventually he guessed what I had done because I kept saying to him that I was saying goodbye as he would be better off without me. During that conversation, I suddenly switched from being 100% sure I had done the right thing to feeling petrified at what I had done. Tony went to tell the nursing staff what he suspected I had done: they told him (I later learned) that it had been my choice to overdose and that they were not going to call an ambulance, but if he wanted to take me to hospital that was up to him. Tony, as you can imagine, was horrified by their attitude and straight away put me in his car and took me to the nearest Accident and Emergency Department. The hospital was a 20-minute drive away, during which I was continually sick. I felt awful – not only physically ill but completely at my wits' end. I was admitted to a ward at the General Hospital and for three days was hooked up to drips. During those days I was ignored by the nursing staff and was later told that 'self-harmers' were frowned upon in the NHS as it was considered attention-seeking behaviour and a drain on resources. In fact Tony later told me that it was not certain that they would even give me the medicine required to counteract my overdose. I was certainly made to feel like a second-class citizen and I vividly remember thinking that if they knew just how desperate and depressed I felt, they couldn't possibly see it as attention-seeking. However, no one asked me how I felt – in fact no was even prepared to listen to why I had done it: they just judged me for what I had done without knowing the facts. Even after three days, when I went back to Warren Abbot I still felt sick all the time and very fragile.

My psychiatrist continued to be nice and supportive and put no pressure on me to leave before I felt well enough. I got the impression that he knew what a bad place my head was in and that he really wanted to help me. At least I had someone on my side.

The dietician that I had been seeing for the last three years sometimes came to visit me at the hospital, but although it was nice to see her I continued to be petrified about what she would think of my weight gain. I thought that others would judge me in the same way I judged myself –with revulsion.

I started doing some Art Therapy once a week, which I liked a great deal, and I also continued with my other art work. I had a lot more spare time than I had ever had at Forest Field. I made a friend with a fellow patient (who was suffering with chronic depression) who I totally clicked with and with whom I kept in contact with for a further 14 years. She became my 'soulmate' and the only person I was able to be totally honest with. I felt that I could tell her anything without her ever judging me and I hoped that she felt the same way about me.

One therapy class that I was offered, but continually turned down, was a fitness class. I felt that I was too big for exercise to have any benefit and had also got to the point where I just couldn't be bothered any more. Controlling my weight had just become too much of a struggle – I was worn out with the constant battle. I was also a little scared that if I did do the exercise class, I would once again become obsessed with exercise – and that in itself was too exhausting to even think about.

It was decided that when I left Warren Abbot I would start seeing a support worker once a week, as well as continuing to regularly see my Community Psychiatric Nurse. During my stay at the hospital I met my support worker for the first time. She was lovely, sweet and kind and I liked her straight away. She continued to work with me for the following eight years.

My depression slowly began to lift during the time I was in this hospital – I even had times when I laughed and I began to enjoy certain things such as chatting with fellow patients and playing board games together or watching TV (which I hadn't experienced for such a long time). I began to think about life outside hospital and about six months after being admitted I felt I was ready to leave. My psychiatrist agreed and so I was discharged. That became my last stay as an inpatient in a psychiatric hospital; I was 31 years old.

CHAPTER 10
Distractions

I left Warren Abbot Hospital and was once again treated in the community. Every week I saw my Community Psychiatric Nurse and my support worker. I rarely saw my psychiatrist and stopped seeing my dietician completely (I'm not sure whose decision that was).

After leaving the hospital, the first thing I realised was how unfit I had become during the previous six months. I was unable to even walk down the road without my legs aching and I had to constantly stop for a breather. I couldn't believe that I had allowed myself to get so unfit. I had gone from being totally obsessed with exercise, swimming up to five miles a day, to being a complete slob whose only exercise over the last six months had been to move from a chair in the lounge at the hospital to a chair in the smoking room. For years I had been a heavy smoker, but during my stay there I smoked at least forty a day. Nearly all the patients seemed to smoke and the main place for socialising was always the smoking room (I finally gave up smoking in 2011).

My mood improved as I left the hospital but I was still obsessed with feelings of revulsion for my body and was constantly overwhelmed with negative thoughts. I also found that I was still getting panic attacks when I went outside. As that was the case every time I went into a supermarket, my support worker started to come shopping with me every week. Once I had got over the shame of her seeing what I had put in my trolley, I found her help worthwhile and my confidence slowly began to grow. Eventually I didn't feel that I was going to have a panic attack every time I went to Sainsbury's. My support worker continued to shop with me every week for the next two years until I was able shop on my own without panicking.

Even though I was repulsed by the way I looked and the amount I weighed, I seemed to no longer possess the willpower to restrict my food intake. I found that difficult to understand but I now believe, years later, that the reason for that lack of willpower was due to God intervening in my life, so that the choice was taken out of my hands (more will be explained about that later).

Not long after leaving Warren Abbot, I decided to buy a puppy. There were a number of reasons for this: I have compassion for all animals (which was the only thing I ever liked about myself.) I felt that I would never allow a pet dog of mine to suffer by not taking it for walks – so I saw that as a way to get over my agoraphobia. I also thought that by becoming a 'mum' to a puppy it would divert my thoughts away from myself to the dog. Bella, the rescue dog I had briefly adopted the year before, had been quite 'damaged' by her previous owners, but I thought that if I got a puppy I could start afresh with training etc. So, after seeing an advertisement in the local paper, I went armed with my £350 and bought an eight-week-old Cocker Spaniel who I named Ted. No one in my family was pleased about my decision. I think they all thought it was a disaster waiting to happen (and who could blame them with my track record?) I am sure they thought that I would never be able to look after him properly, but for 14 years I had him as my constant companion. Ted died in 2014, which was heart breaking. Throughout his life he hadn't had the best health (mainly inbred problems), which meant that he had to have a lot of nursing, but I have no doubt that he nursed / helped me just as much as I hope I did him.

After a couple of months of having Ted, I slowly got over my agoraphobia and began to meet lots of 'doggy walkers' who became good friends. We all had something in common, which was that we all loved dogs. Very rarely did I ever have to talk about myself because the conversation was always about our dogs. By having Ted in my life, I began to have structure and routine and I knew that if I lost weight again he would suffer. When I got him, I already had two cats. I was so fortunate that my lodger at the time had always been prepared to look after the cats (Arnold and Cleo) when I was in hospital. I soon found that the loyalty and dependence of a dog meant a totally different relationship than with the cats. They were, however, all 'my family' and it did me so much good to feel that I was caring for them and that they were relying on me to stay well. I hoped that Ted and the cats would live happily together and although Arnold quickly accommodated Ted, Cleo was scared stiff of him. For Cleo's sake I therefore had to keep Ted and her apart with a stairgate in the hallway.

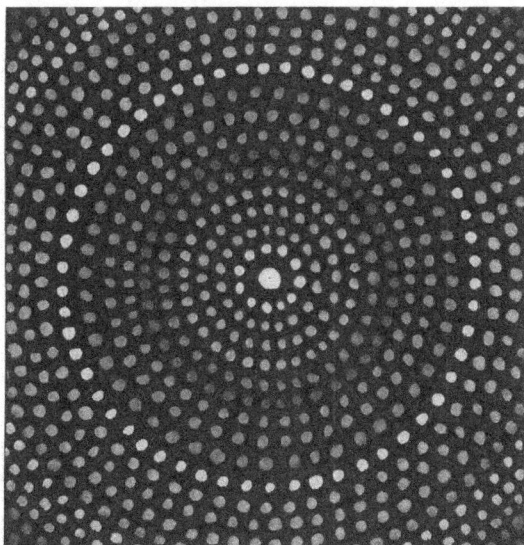

My thoughts and actions are getting more and more intense, spiralling out of control

I continued to get an income from sickness benefits and income support and was able to live solely on that money. I continued to have a relationship with Tony and saw him two or three times a week. I did, however, still avoid social situations. It was clear that I had developed a 'social phobia' over the years and would do anything to find excuses not to go to social gatherings. With Tony, though, we would often go to pubs and go shopping together and I slowly began to get glimpses of what normal life was like. I also began to allow him to hug me even though I still wasn't totally happy about it.

During the years following my discharge from Warren Abbot, I began to get hooked on going to coffee shops. I would walk into town (to attempt to keep my weight down) then reward myself with a café latte, have a read of my book and then walk back home again. It was my idea of bliss. I hadn't ever read a book by choice before that time, but was now able to concentrate better and found that I really enjoyed reading. I discovered that by totally immersing myself in a book I stopped thinking my usual negative thoughts. The time I used to spend drawing I now spent reading.

So, during the eight years between 2000 and 2008, I continued to just 'plod along'. My depression was generally better than it had been, but at times I still felt very 'down.' I didn't really see a future for myself that was any different to that. I just lived day by day as best as I could.

CHAPTER 11

A Light Bulb Moment

In late December 2007 and early January 2008, I suddenly realised that I no longer wanted to die – in fact not only did I not want to die, but I wanted to enjoy life again. I also found myself realising that there was more to life than continual dieting. It really was a 'light bulb' moment. It was as if someone had turned on the light which lifted me from the darkness that had enveloped me for so many years.

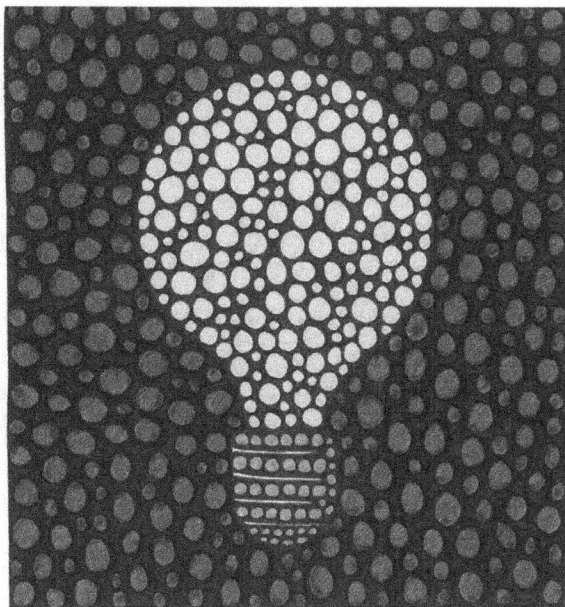

At that time of sudden realisation, I began to see a future for myself and Tony and we began to discuss getting married. It was the first time that I had been well enough to contemplate our future together and we decided that we should start planning our wedding. By then, we had been in a relationship for 17 years and although it wasn't always what you could call a 'normal' relationship, we both knew each other extremely well and wanted to take our relationship further.

In early February, Tony and I went to London for a mini-break. On our way back we were both astounded at how mild the weather was for that time of year. Tony dropped me off at my house and then went home. Just as I was settling down to have a little nap after our exhausting few days, I got a phone call from Tony pleading with me to meet him down at the beach near his house. I really didn't want to go as I was exhausted, but 30 minutes later Ted (the dog) and I met up with him. We walked along the beach to some large rocks. We had previously affectionately called those rocks 'our rocks' as we often sat and chatted on them. The weather was surreal – it was February yet the sun was so strong and it felt like a gorgeous summer's day. While sitting on 'our rocks' chatting, Tony suddenly got down on one knee and proposed to me. It didn't come as a complete surprise as we had been speaking about getting married for weeks, but I had given up on him ever proposing to me because he seemed to be taking so long. I was very pleased to accept and that beach has now become an even more special place for both of us.

We made arrangements to meet up with the vicar at the church where Tony had been worshipping for the previous twelve years. The meetings weren't totally straightforward because Tony had been married before, so we had to go through two pretty tough interviews before being given the go-ahead to get married in the church. The date for the wedding was set for 9 August 2008.

Even though my depression had lifted, I was still struggling with anxiety. I had what the medical profession called 'generalised anxiety', which meant that I was in a permanently frantic state almost always accompanied by physical symptoms. I decided that because of the way I felt, I couldn't cope with the stress of organising a wedding - so Tony volunteered to do it all (organising people had always been his forte). Initially I felt a huge sense of relief but it soon became evident that Tony was organising the type of wedding I really didn't want. For example, he wanted 450 people at the evening reception and 300 at the church service – I only knew about 50 of those people and began to realise that at my own wedding I would only know a handful of people. The reason he wanted such a large wedding was because he had lived in the area for a long time and knew a large number of people: he wanted them all to celebrate our special day. I had lived the life of a recluse for the past ten years and had lost a lot of friends in the process, so it was no surprise that I didn't know many of the people that over these years had become Tony's friends.

Tony also began to talk about things we would and wouldn't do when we were married. I became scared that he was going to be controlling and that, coupled with the wedding plans that I didn't want, meant I had second thoughts about getting married: I called off the engagement. The week following that decision was horrendous for both of us. I was in turmoil about whether I had made the correct decision and every time I spoke to Tony it would end in awful arguments. As that week went on, I began to realise that I couldn't imagine my life without Tony being a part of it: and I missed him terribly. He felt the same way, so after a week of being 'unengaged', the wedding was back on. We discussed the fact that the wedding was not the type I wanted but I realised that it was what Tony wanted, so I went along with it. I tried to be laid back about it, but the worry of walking down the aisle hardly knowing anyone became overwhelming. I could not envisage being able to do it without having a panic attack.

The one thing that I did have to organise myself was my wedding dress and the bridesmaid dresses. My four nieces were to be my bridesmaids. They were 2, 4, 8 and 13 years old, so would look very sweet. Mum visited for the day in February and we went to the bridal shop in my nearby town. I tried on a couple of dresses but neither of them made me look particularly special. The third one I tried on was a different story – I knew straight away that it was the right one. Mum told me that day, when we left the shop, that I looked beautiful and although I was so chuffed with her comment, I did feel angry that the first time she had ever said that to me was when I was buying my wedding dress at 39 years of age. She has also never said it since. Despite those feelings, we both remained in a good mood and although the dress was rather pricey (Mum offered to pay for it) I was jubilant. I remember walking arm in arm with her when we left the bridal shop, feeling the closest I had ever felt to her. I felt so positive that day - I had always been afraid that I wouldn't look nice in any dress that I tried on, but now I was sure that Tony would really like the dress and hopefully feel proud of me.

I still occasionally saw my psychiatrist at the local adult mental health clinic and I told him how scared I was about the wedding. He prescribed some new drugs, but the side-effects were so awful that even with only five days left before my wedding, I was convinced I was going to be too ill to turn up at the church. I decided to stop those new drugs and to go back on my old ones and to rely on the Valium that he had given me to get through the day.

When we had decided to get married back in the beginning of January, I hadn't really been too fussed if I got married in a church or in a registry office. However, Tony was adamant that he wanted to get married in his church and when we got the go-ahead from the vicar, I knew that the time had come for me to look into the Christian faith in more detail. I didn't want to be hypocritical by going along with the church service with very little knowledge of Christianity and what it all meant. For years Tony had nagged me to take part in an Alpha Course and although I had in the past started, but not finished one, now seemed the ideal opportunity to try to complete a whole course. I was now able to concentrate, and I also had an interest - so I felt ready to start one at a nearby church with Tony coming along to support me. It was a ten-week course starting off with a meal each evening (which had for so many years terrified me) followed by a talk and then small group discussions with an opportunity for questions and answers. Apart from initial nerves, I soon enjoyed the course and made some friends. Although I found everything I learnt interesting and believable, I can't say it changed my life.

During this Alpha Course, there was the opportunity to say a prayer to invite Jesus into your life. I had already said that prayer at the beginning of January after Tony had given me a booklet called 'Why Jesus?' and although I wasn't totally committed to Christianity at that time, I had thought 'what have I got to lose by saying it?' As soon as I had said the prayer (sitting on my bed on my own in the house) I had a weird sensation and was 'tingling' all over. I remember thinking to myself whether it was possible that God had heard my prayer and that was why I had had this tingling sensation. Although that was amazing, I soon put it to the back of my mind and didn't experience anything like it while on the Alpha Course. Since saying that prayer, I considered myself a Christian, but didn't really know how to progress from there. I also felt much more comfortable about getting married in a church and Tony was over the moon that I had at last completed the course. We often had discussions about aspects of Christianity and faith and it was very handy to have him answer my questions (which he was always able to do).

Before I knew it, the day of our wedding was here.

CHAPTER 12

A Strange Emotion

As soon as I awoke on the morning of the wedding, I felt a complete peace about the day. It was such a different feeling to how I had felt in the months leading up to that day. I did have my Valium at the ready just in case I got too anxious, but after having my hair done at the local salon in the morning, I knew that I didn't need to take it. My Mum has since told me that she was convinced my anxiety would get the better of me and dreaded what that would mean. I think she was as amazed at how calm I was that morning, especially as the weather was the worst you could possibly imagine with heavy rain and gale force winds forecast to last all day.

The wedding car arrived at my house at 2.30pm ready to take Dad and me to the church for 3pm. When we arrived, a very kind man - who at the time I did not know - came out to meet me with a huge umbrella and managed to keep me clean and dry while I got into the church.

By the time I arrived, everyone was already seated and when I saw the number of people there, I was stunned that so many would want to be part of our wedding day. As I walked down the aisle with my Dad at the start of the ceremony, I didn't really mind that there were faces I didn't recognise. Things that had frightened the life out of me leading up to that day, such as saying my vows, just weren't a problem at all and I can honestly say that I have never before experienced how I felt that day. I was so confident and really felt like a princess. I didn't think I would ever experience those two feelings in my lifetime.

Because of the awful weather, photographs were taken inside the church, instead of in the grounds as planned. Family and close friends then made their way to a restaurant for a sit-down meal. This proved to be a great success and then there were only the speeches left. As my Dad was making his way up to do his 'father of the bride' speech, I felt panicky because I did not have a clue about what he was going to say about me. I really hoped it would be similar to other 'father of the bride' speeches I had heard, in which the father always says how lucky he is to have such a lovely daughter and how her new husband is such a lucky man. My father said nothing about that: instead he talked at length about how, if I had persevered at hockey and not given up, I could have been in the England squad. Once again, my parents made it clear that not only had I never stuck at anything, but also that I had let everyone down. If my Dad couldn't sing my praises even on my wedding day, then it was never going to happen. That made me really sad and also made me feel that my parents did not, in fact, feel lucky to have a daughter like me. It reinforced what I had thought for years: that their love for me wasn't the same as the love other parents have for their children.

However, it was nice to hear my brother later tell me that he had found the church service really emotional, mainly because it was obvious that I had moved on from being so ill for so long.

After we had finished in the restaurant, we went to the local Community Centre where another 450 people were waiting to celebrate the evening reception with us. My nerves then set in because I knew the 'first dance' was looming. I wanted to do a normal slow dance (like most others do) but Tony insisted we did some fancy routine that we had been rehearsing for the previous few weeks and which was much against my wishes. The problem was that the dance was too complicated for me and made me anxious in case I looked an idiot. After that dance was over it meant that I could relax for the rest of the evening.

As the end of the evening approached Tony and I left for a local hotel. It had been an amazing day; I couldn't have dreamt of it going any better but already it was a blur and I felt that I wanted to go through it all again so that I could take more of it in.

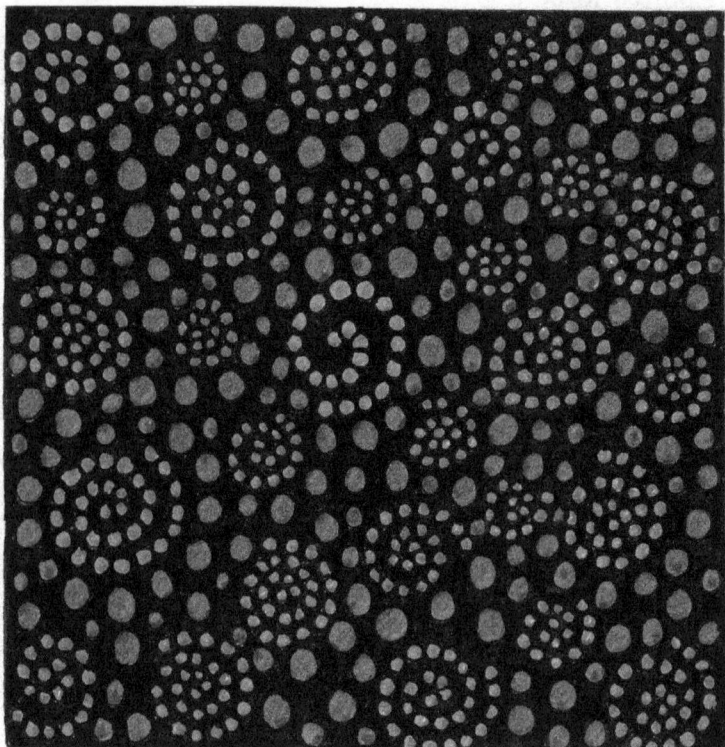

All my thoughts are so muddled, as if my head is spinning

The next morning, after meeting with family over breakfast, Tony and I left for our honeymoon. We were off to Rome for three days and then on to Florence for another three days. We were both really looking forward to our honeymoon and on the journey to the airport I remember not quite believing that I was now married. I now had to get used to being called by my new surname and also get used to calling Tony 'my husband.'

We arrived in Rome and stayed in the most amazing hotel. We were shown to our room and then went straight out for dinner as we were starving. On our return to the hotel, the reception desk called us over and told us that we had been upgraded to not only a better room, but to a suite which turned out to be the best in the hotel. The ceiling looked like something out of the Sistine Chapel; we were both blown away with how spoilt we felt. We had a fantastic time in Rome but our time there went too quickly and before we knew it we were making our way to Florence by train, travelling First Class. On arriving at our new hotel, which was gorgeous and in a fantastic location, we realised that once again we had been given another top-class suite. I felt like I was in a dream and with champagne in our room on our arrival, I felt so spoilt and special.

We both vowed that we would go back to the two hotels in five years' time. Unfortunately, that has not yet happened and in reality we might never be able to afford it. We were both so blessed on our honeymoon and it really was a very special time for us - one that we will never forget.

When we returned back to England six days later, I was due to move into Tony's house and the plan was to rent out my old house. Since we were both keen that our marital home would feel like 'our home' rather than 'Tony's home', quite a lot of renovations were being done which weren't finished by the time we got back from Italy. So we decided that I would delay moving in with him until that work was completed and the house no longer resembled a building site. Three weeks later I moved in - with Ted the dog and Arnold the cat. Before we got married we discussed how it would not be fair to move Cleo to Tony's house with the way she felt about Ted. I knew a lovely older lady who had recently lost her own cat and who was keen to adopt Cleo; now 13 years old. Arnold was 17 and Ted was eight years old when we moved to Tony's house. When we finally moved in Tony even insisted on carrying me over the threshold, much to my amusement. I soon realised our new house looked amazing; some walls had been knocked down and after we had bought new furniture the house really did feel like home.

CHAPTER 13

Bad News

Even though I had virtually no anxiety on my wedding day, generalised anxiety continued to be a big issue in my life. Every day I would experience its physical symptoms, but was not always aware of what exactly I was worrying about. It seemed that just 'everyday life' caused me anxiety. I was still unable to work because of this disability, but now that I was married and had moved to a new area, I no longer had any help from the mental health service. I'd had help from them since 1996 but was no longer regarded as ill enough to warrant further help, especially as a lot of services were being cut. Although I was petrified about no longer receiving support and worried about changing to a new GP who would be unaware of my past, I did feel relieved about no longer having to attend appointments to discuss my 'feelings'. After twelve years of therapy, I'd had enough, but I also realised that there was very little more they could do for me.

Once I had moved into our new marital home, Tony agreed to let me change the garden to how I wanted it - to my mind it closely resembled an overgrown rubbish dump and seriously needed some TLC. I liked gardening, but my old house had a very small plot so there was a limit to how much I could do. Soon gardening became a real passion and I had great plans for what I wanted to do. I found that gardening allowed me to 'escape' from any bad thoughts and I relished seeing the plants develop from small shoots into well-established shrubs. I also loved doing small projects of landscape gardening and achieving good results - all by myself.

During our first year of marriage I decided that, as I had got married in church, I needed to develop my faith from the little I had gained from the Alpha Course of the year before. I therefore decided that I would begin to go to church regularly, but the problem was that I didn't feel comfortable at the church in which Tony and I were married. The morning service that Tony had always attended had an enormous congregation of about 300 people. Everyone knew me there as 'Tony's wife' rather than as myself and because of my anxiety about going to crowded places, I decided to try the church in which I had completed my Alpha Course. Tony and I had already joined a home group from that church and so it seemed the natural place for me to try. Although I really learnt a lot from the sermons, I didn't feel comfortable worshipping in a different church to Tony - and I somehow felt bad about not going to the church we were married in, especially as Tony really loved it. So I decided to give the church another chance, and slowly began to feel more at home there. In 2009 I started to go to the evening service which I found to be more to my liking, especially as the congregation was much smaller. The evening service had a very different atmosphere with fewer distractions, such as babies crying. I soon felt much closer to God at those services and it became my regular worship time. Tony continued to attend the morning service, but he also came to most of evening services with me.

In 2009, Tony and I decided to try for a baby. I had never felt particularly maternal, but realised my time was running out as I was now 41 years old and it was a case of now or never. Amazingly I became pregnant the first time we tried and we were over the moon. Although Tony had two grown-up children from his previous marriage and was 19 years older than me, he was so looking forward to going through the whole experience again.

Everything started off fine, but I soon became aware of how anxious I was about the pregnancy. I had to stop taking my anti-depressant and anti-psychotic drugs, which really concerned me. I had an overwhelming fear that something awful was going to happen to the baby and that I was going to lose it. When I started having morning sickness, my anxiety levels increased and most of the time I felt ill.

I was booked in for my first scan at 12 weeks and had seen the midwife the week before. Two days before the scan, I started to bleed and after ringing the hospital I was told to go straight for a scan. The threat of losing the baby was suddenly very real. When the nurse performed the scan, I knew I had lost the baby because she asked for a consultant to come in and give his opinion. Although they could see the baby, there was no heartbeat and Tony and I were given the horrible news. We were also told that because of the size of the baby it had died in week seven, whereas now it was week 12. I was distraught that I had been carrying a dead baby for the last five weeks. I was told that I would either miscarry naturally, or in case that didn't happen, I was booked in for a 'D and C' ten days later. I was also told that I was still getting morning sickness because my body thought I was still pregnant.

Both of us were devastated. Tony had been so excited about having a baby that he had told literally the whole world, so now he had the horrible task of telling everyone that I had lost the baby. Over the next two days, my body began the process of miscarrying naturally, which was traumatic.

I began to feel real anger towards God for allowing the miscarriage to happen. I couldn't understand why, when things were going so well, that it had happened. As I was certain that God had done an amazing job at healing me, I couldn't understand what was going on and seriously began to question my faith. I stopped going to church over the following few months and even though Tony tried to discuss that maybe I had lost the baby for a reason, I felt so angry and couldn't even acknowledge that there was indeed a God.

As the pain and hurt subsided over the next few months I slowly returned to church and came round to Tony's way of thinking - I had probably lost the baby for a reason.

We should have started to try for another baby at that stage, but somehow I couldn't face the fear of another miscarriage and as there was no guarantee that that wouldn't be the case, we just never tried. Looking back now many years later, and no longer able to conceive, I do feel really sad about never having had children. Considering how ill I was with anorexia, I have always been amazed that apparently I haven't had any long-term health problems. However, I do feel that if I hadn't been ill for such a long time, I would have got married to Tony at a much younger age and almost certainly would have had kids. So in a way, I feel quite fortunate that not having children is the only lasting effect I have had from suffering with anorexia. Slowly, after returning to church, my faith again grew.

In September 2010 Tony and I were invited to help out leading a group on the forthcoming Alpha Course at our local church. Although feeling inadequate I agreed, on the condition that Tony was the leader and I was his assistant (whose main role was to make the others feel at ease). I was anxious about it, but forced myself to take part and soon got to realise how lovely our group of participants were. Not only that, but by participating in the Alpha Course again and being in a totally different place than when I attended the first course (when I was somewhat cynical in my attitude) I gained so much more the second time around. I soon made fantastic new friends, and our 'group' went on to complete the 'Beta Course' before forming a home group together.

In the summer of 2011 my faith had continued to grow and so I decided it was time to renew my baptism vows (I was first christened as a child). Being an adult this time around, I wanted to make a public declaration about how important God had become in my life. After He helped me through so much, in order to get better from my years of mental health issues, I felt that the time was right to publicly thank Him. I began to feel uneasy about being a smoker and a Christian, so I tried to give up for the umpteenth time. However, this time was very different to all my other attempts:

every time I had a craving, I decided to pray for help to resist those cravings. By the time of my baptism, it had been 10 weeks since my last cigarette.

It was decided that my baptism would take place in the sea and on 4 September I was baptised by full submersion. It was the most amazing experience and one that I will never forget. The only regret I had was that I felt I couldn't invite my family because I felt they would mock me and think that I had 'cracked up' and joined some sort of cult. Even though our church was Anglican, it was so far out of their comfort zone that they would never have understood why I wanted to be baptised a second time.

As part of the baptism procedure, I was asked to write a testimony about why I had decided to get baptised and explain my journey in making that decision. This was to be publicly read out, so all those that were there could hear about the journey and hopefully be encouraged. I was being baptised with four others and there were about 150 people who had come to support us, so that in itself was quite frightening. During this testimony (which you can read in Appendix 3) I mentioned my illness over the years and how I had eventually got better due to God's help.

The thought of reading out 'My Testimony' to so many people was scary, especially as most of them didn't have a clue that I used to be ill. I was worried that I might be judged, and that after reading it out I would have no secrets left, so inevitably I thought I would feel very vulnerable. However, the response I got afterwards was so positive that it allayed all my fears. The curate who helped baptise me even told me afterwards that my testimony was one of the most powerful he had ever heard - so this too made it all worthwhile. I hoped that others would see that we can never give up hope that God can and will do amazing things in our lives.

All in all, the whole experience was amazing. I felt confident reading out my testimony (another 'God moment') and I knew that reaffirming my baptism vows was the right thing to do. A week later I decided to give my Dad a copy of my testimony. I regret to say that he never commented on it and I don't even know if he showed it to my Mum. Because my Dad did not make a comment, I knew I had done the right thing by not inviting my family – I didn't want anything to spoil what turned into such a special time for me.

The time had come for me to think seriously about getting a job, but I was still sometimes crippled with symptoms from my anxiety. I wasn't sure how my nerves would cope with a job involving meeting new people; I still suffered from a lack of self-esteem and confidence. The only thing that I was qualified to do was teach PE, but I was adamant I didn't want the stress of working as a secondary school teacher again and wondered whether anyone would employ me, as I hadn't worked since 1998. I still had some friends who were teachers at the school I used to work in and although they had loved their jobs, they now complained of the increased levels of stress that teaching was causing. Not one of them could recommend going back to teaching and it wasn't something I really wanted to do anyway.

Even if I didn't return to teaching, I knew my anxiety had to improve before I could seriously consider getting any type of job - I had the physical symptoms of anxiety on a daily basis. The last thing I wanted was to start a job only to have to give it up a few weeks after starting. Fortunately there was no immediate need, as Tony had always made it clear that he would support me financially until I felt the time was right to start working again.

Just before Christmas 2012 I was going through a particularly difficult time – I felt that my anxiety was becoming out of control, which led me to feel quite low. I had this fear that things were beginning to again overwhelm me and I was beginning to feel depressed. I decided that the best course of action would be to go on a three-day retreat so I could focus entirely on asking God to help me. I seemed unable to do that while I was at home. I had always wanted to go on a retreat and now seemed the perfect opportunity. I booked to go to Testament Sanctuary in East Sussex for two nights, but also decided that I would also pop into the Fountain of Love

House on the way, which I knew was holding a healing service on the morning I was travelling. I had been recommended this place by church friends, but also Tony had been there a year before with a very ill friend of ours.

After a very long drive, I arrived at the healing service feeling nervous because I had no idea what to expect. After being there for five minutes I realised what an amazing place it was and learnt that they held weekend healing retreats once a month. After the service I was invited to stay for lunch and I knew that I had to book a place to go on one of their weekends. I hoped it would be possible for me to get healing for my anxiety problem - after all, God had already done so much for me. Although I would have loved to have stayed longer, I had to leave to go to Testament Sanctuary, a short distance away, where I was booked in. During my time there I spent a lot of time praying and was able to leave a few days later feeling refreshed and renewed after spending time with God. I felt more at peace with myself and was able to get into perspective that which had previously overwhelmed me. While I was there, Mum happened to ring and was shocked when I told her where I was. She was convinced that the only reason I was there was because Tony and I were about to split up. I assured her we weren't and tried to explain how I had felt leading up to this point and how it was a positive thing that I now recognised when worries were overwhelming me and hence could do something about them. I'm not sure she was convinced so I had to ring her again on my return home to reassure her that Tony and I weren't getting divorced.

Even though I had a rewarding time at Testament Sanctuary, I knew that if there was any hope of getting better from my chronic anxiety I would have to return to the Fountain of Love House for a weekend healing retreat. Once I got home, I booked a place for six weeks later. During my time there we had teaching, services, quiet times and prayer with the prayer ministry team. It was an amazing experience and one that I will never forget. However, for the month following my stay there, nothing changed with my anxiety issues and I began to give up hope that I would ever be totally well. I knew that God chooses if and when to heal, but I was still disappointed that nothing appeared to have changed with my anxiety. However, over the following two years I realised that my generalised anxiety was definitely improving and I continued to have reduced symptoms right up to 2015 when my life once again took a turn for the worse. I explain more about this in Chapter 15.

During the years 2012 and 2013, some friends had mentioned to me that I would make a good counsellor. They said that I was a good listener and people - sometimes strangers - seemed to always be able to open up to me. In all the time that I was ill with anorexia and depression, I was always desperate to speak to someone who had recovered to give me hope that it was indeed possible, but also to know that the feelings I was having were not completely unheard of. I always felt that I was completely on my own with all my thoughts and struggles. It would have meant so much to me to have been able to talk to someone who had recovered, but alas that never happened. After my friends' comments I began to wonder if, because I had gone through so much - anorexia, depression, anxiety, self-harm, suicidal thoughts, agoraphobia, and a touch of OCD - that I would have empathy for others and would be able to use my experiences to help them. I started to look into counselling training. All my years of being counselled had not helped me and it was not until God became a part of my life that things massively improved. So I began to think about Christian Counselling training and enquired of the training centre in Surrey where Christian counselling originated. After attending a five-day Introduction to Biblical Counselling course in 2012 I began to seriously consider whether this was something I wanted to do. I decided, with the encouragement of friends, to apply for a place on the Christian Counselling course and in May 2013 I was awarded a place to start in the summer of that year.

There were a couple of factors that worried me about the course. Firstly, it meant that one weekend a month I would be in residential training and secondly there would be assignments and exams. Exams had always worried me as I was always rubbish at them.

At the same time as applying for a place on the training course, I started a new job: the first job I had had in 16 years. My new job was coaching PE to primary school children. It was for three afternoons a week and therefore suited me down to the ground. I felt nervous and very rusty about teaching / coaching again, but thought it wouldn't have the same pressures that a normal teaching job would have. It was fantastic to be working and feel a valued member of society again and I loved having the extra money. The only drawback was that I was teaching / coaching in a difficult school. The staff weren't friendly and a lot of the children had behavioural problems. So it was not as easy as I had hoped, but it did pay well and I really had no other options open to me.

After I had been working at the school for about a month, I had an accident. I was playing a game of 'tag' as a warm-up game with a class of six-year-olds, when my right leg locked as I was running, causing me to fall over - straight away it was obvious I had injured my knee very badly.

I eventually discovered, after having an MRI scan, that I had torn my medial ligament and completely ruptured my anterior cruciate ligament. I then had an eight-month wait before undergoing knee reconstruction surgery. Unfortunately, as I didn't know when I was going to have the operation, I had to make the hard decision to defer my counselling training for a year. To pass the course I had to have a 100% attendance, so I couldn't risk starting and having to take time off for the operation and rehab. Even though that was a hard decision to make, the college were very understanding and agreed that I could start in September 2014 instead.

I was also unable to continue with my PE job until months after the operation (so I was out for almost a year). I found it confusing why, when once again things seemed to be going so well for me, that the injury put such a 'spanner in the works'. I did my utmost not to keep thinking about why God had allowed the injury to happen. Maybe He thought that I wasn't quite ready to start the counselling training? I was quite shocked at how 'down' I became in that year of being injured, especially during the long wait for my operation. As I wasn't working, once again I felt that I wasn't a valued member of society and that I had failed with the counselling training before I had even started.

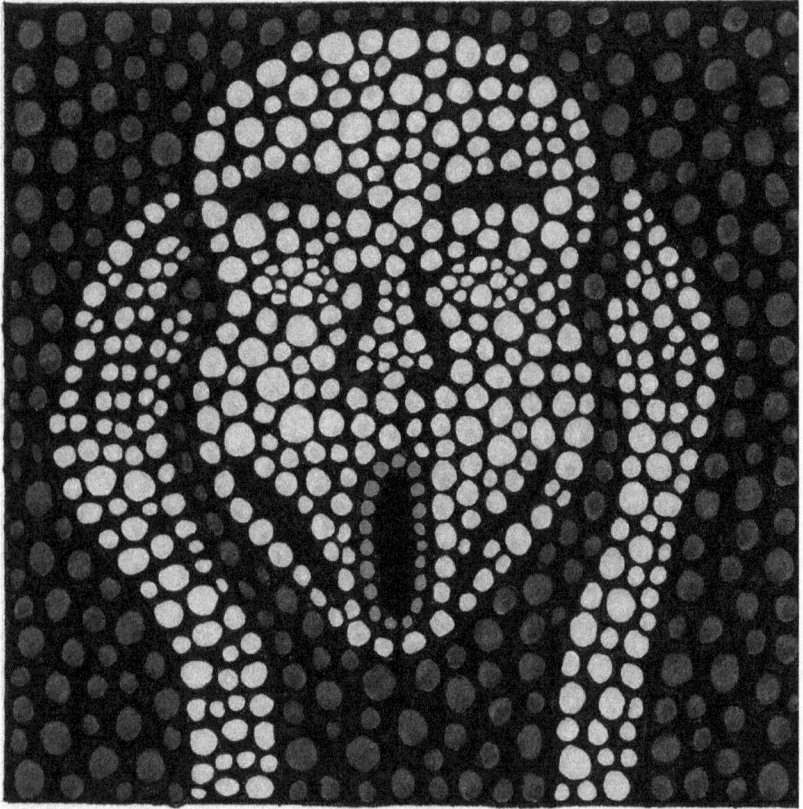

So many guilty feelings: how do I cope with them?

In January 2014 I eventually had my knee reconstruction. I had months of physio ahead and, as I had no definite date to go back to work, it was the ideal opportunity to get my memories and experiences all down on paper so I didn't go stir-crazy sitting at home twiddling my thumbs.

My depression lifted as I began to focus on this book, but it made me realise how any 'bad' event can trigger a bout of depression. The year in which, because of being in pain, I had been unable to do what I wanted, had hit me really hard - much more than I expected. I now realise that what affects one person may affect another person totally differently and also that any sequence of events can trigger 'bad times'. The constant encouragement from my husband to get on and write this book allowed me to focus on other things and thank goodness lifted me from being 'down in the dumps' ... until the time I discovered I needed many more operations on my knee. In the summer of this year Ted died and both Tony and I were devastated. We knew he was getting older and that the time was near, but it still was such a loss to us. I cried for weeks as he had been my constant companion for nearly 14 years and I now had nothing to focus on except all the trauma that was happening with my knee. After losing Ted, my depression got a lot worse.

CHAPTER 14

Downward Spiral

I was about to conclude this book in 2014 with the 'happy ever after' scenario when everything went horribly wrong. I felt my book was pretty much finished and was about to approach a publisher when two things stopped me.

The first was that I was worried that my parents would get to know about my book, which is critical of how they had treated me. Although I used to feel bitter, I now feel I can forgive them, realising that there were particular reasons why they acted / said what they did; due partly to the way they themselves were brought up and their particular personalities / issues. The aim of this book has always been to try and prevent other parents / carers from making similar mistakes with their child(ren) and loved ones. The aim is also to highlight how someone with anorexia, body dysmorphia and / or low self-esteem thinks and feels in certain situations or/and at certain times.

The second was that, in 2015-2018, my life was suddenly turned upside-down. Following my injury and subsequent six operations, I suddenly found myself spiralling back to an anorexic way of life. I felt it would be hypocritical to take my book any further when I had previously implied that I was fully recovered. After much discussion with Tony, I decided that instead of being hypocritical I would instead highlight the need to not be complacent and understand that a traumatic event or situation can potentially tip one back over the edge. I now believe that it is more realistic to see myself not as 'fully recovered' from anorexia but instead to be 'in remission'.

Over the following chapters I will describe what tipped me back into anorexic behaviour; some 15 years since my previous relapse.

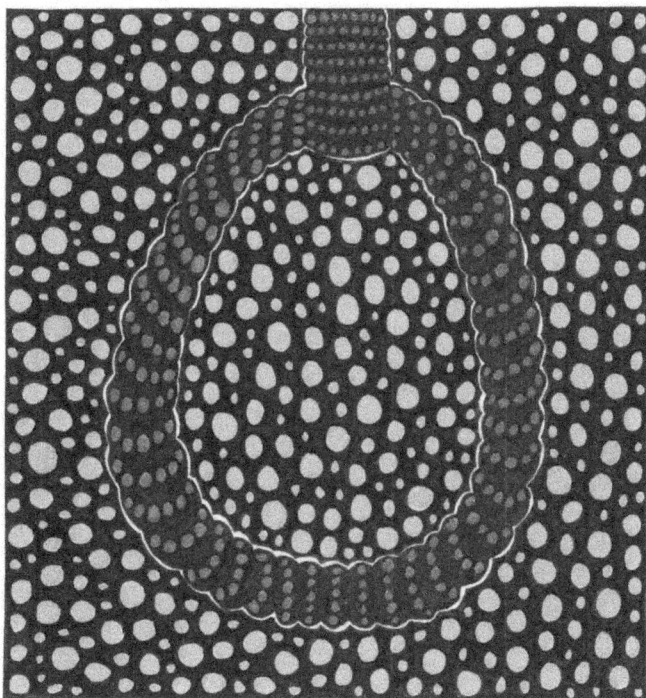

Desperation

CHAPTER 15

Please Help Me!

ollowing my knee reconstruction operation in January 2014 and after months of physiotherapy, it became clear that I wasn't progressing as well as others in my weekly physio class. I kept hoping that if I continued with my exercises it would happen; I just needed to remain patient. In 2015, however, I was in the same position as I was the year before. I still had a very painful knee that prevented me from doing very much. I therefore decided to make an appointment with another consultant and after a further MRI scan, I was told I needed another operation to fix the problem. So, I had a second operation and then began another round of rehab, but with a new physiotherapist. Nevertheless, after six months I was feeling increasingly concerned as my knee felt worse than ever. I therefore made a follow-up private appointment with the surgeon who had carried out my second operation.

During the appointment the consultant was far from the charming self he had been before operating on me and very soon made it clear that he was irritated that I had returned to see him because my knee was no better. The last thing he said was that he could do no more for me. I left the hospital in shock and was inconsolable. All I could think was that I had put all my trust in this surgeon but had been left with a knee that didn't function properly and which still caused me so much pain. I couldn't stop crying as I drove home and could hardly see the road through my tears. This was the start of my downward spiral back to an anorexic way of life.

When I arrived back home, I told Tony what the consultant had said to me. Neither of us could believe that my knee would be this way for the remainder of my life.

The next morning Tony came up with the idea of making an appointment to see a different consultant for a second opinion. The consultant we chose - consultant number three - shared a mutual friend with us and seemed the obvious choice. Tony had met him a few years earlier at one of our friend's dinner parties. After phoning his secretary we were given an appointment a few days later. He turned out to be lovely and was quick to reassure me that further treatment was possible. He suggested I have another MRI scan and said that he would refer me to one of his colleagues who was a knee specialist. In the meantime, the scan showed that I needed a screw surgically removed, which he performed a few weeks later: that was surgery number three.

In May 2016 I finally met the knee specialist who became my new consultant – my fourth - and who continues to treat me to this day. After yet another scan he suggested a further operation: this went ahead and once again I started a long journey of rehab with a new physiotherapist recommended by my consultant.

During this time my depression deepened and my anxiety levels were extreme. It seemed I was going through one trauma after another with my knee and I began to lack trust in the medical profession. I had so many questions about why my knee still hurt, or why it still didn't work as a normal knee. The more I ruminated about everything, the more desperate I became.

By this stage I was massively restricting my food. I felt worthless following how consultant number two had made me feel and I no longer wanted to carry on living. However, I began listening to two songs that Tony had composed: in fact I began listening to them constantly. One was called 'Out Of The Depths' and the other 'If You Call His Name'. You can read the lyrics to these songs at the back of the book. These two Christian songs became my prayers and were my only means of reassurance and comfort during these anxious times.

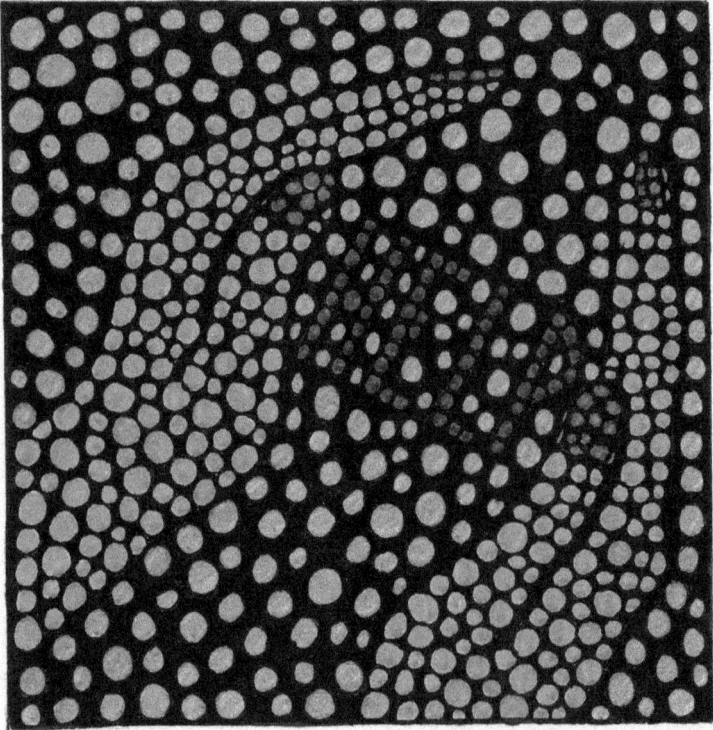

Someone please help me - I'm too
exhausted to fight any more

A year later, and after a lot of physiotherapy I was slowly improving, but needed to have a further screw removed, which became the fifth operation on my knee. I was still restricting my food and was determined to get to a lower weight. I suppose I reverted back to the one thing that made me feel good about myself. I also had the bizarre fear that the consultant would say I was carrying too much weight and that was why my knee still hurt. I also began exercising more than I should, mainly to aid my weight loss. My knee was continually flaring up because I was overdoing it. Because of my knee, the only exercise I could do was swim and walk. I kept using the excuse of swimming being helpful to strengthen the muscles supporting my kneecap, when in fact I was trying desperately to lose more weight. Losing weight was the only thing that made me feel good about myself. In reality I was self-harming once again, as I knew exercising like this would ultimately cause me more pain. Rather absurdly, I felt that I needed to punish myself – I felt useless, worthless, and that my life, as I knew it, was over. I was conscious that I had wasted most of my 20s and 30s with my eating disorder and now coming to terms with being inactive was very difficult.

The final knee surgery I had - operation number six - was in January 2019. Fortunately, this was a fairly minor op that took only a month from which to recover.

Since 2016 I've had amazing orthopaedic surgeons who have helped me tremendously and a fantastic physiotherapist. Nevertheless, despite all their help and compassion I was still having very dark days in 2018. I spotted the warning signs of progressing back to the anorexic way of life but was complacent. I remember saying to myself "I won't let it take control this time" but I failed miserably. I found it impossible to go a day without weighing myself, counting calories and worrying about weight gain.

Back in 2008 I had been diagnosed with Coeliac disease and in 2017 I was diagnosed with a second auto-immune condition called Sjogren's syndrome – a condition that affects parts of the body that produce fluids. This took 18 months to diagnose. I was working at the time but had to have time off for sickness and so claimed Employment and Support Allowance for a year. This felt like such a backward step after being on benefits between 1998 and 2009, and it did my self-worth no good at all. After returning to work, I was then made redundant in 2018 - another event which made me feel completely worthless.

CHAPTER 16
Finding the Key

During this time my anxiety was sky high and it was suggested that I consider attending an internationally known Anxiety Residential Course. My parents kindly paid the course fee and a month later I attended, with Tony as support.

The Anxiety Course showed me that I needed to find some quality of life different from being highly active (over-exercising) and with a new line of work away from sport. I found this very challenging because the only thing I ever felt I had achieved in my life was due to my sporting ability. It was the only thing that had helped my self-esteem.

One suggestion from the Course was to get a new dog, as this would help distract me from focusing on my anxiety. This was something I had dreamt about since Ted had died some five years earlier. Friends often said that I hadn't been the same since Ted's death, so Tony and I decided that this was something we should consider. Tony loved dogs as much as I did and, as he now worked part-time from home and I wasn't working, it seemed the ideal time for us to get a dog.

I had become friends with a woman called Kirsty, who soon made it clear that if we were to stay friends she didn't want to listen to my depressive talk – she wanted to enjoy being out and not end up feeling depressed listening to me. From that moment I realised that if I wanted to continue our friendship I needed to be 'fun' to be with. Although Kirsty's reaction may sound harsh, I do now understand how someone else's depression can drag you down. Kirsty made me laugh a lot (which I hadn't done for years) and showed me how to enjoy life and, as the saying goes, 'laughter is the best form of medicine'.

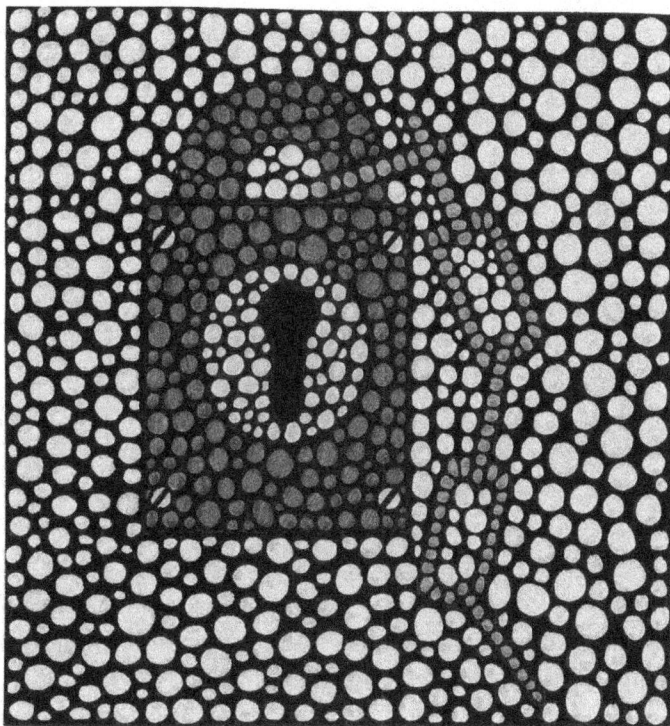

Am I ever going to find the key to solve all the misery I feel?

Around the time that Tony and I were considering what type of dog to get, Kirsty told me that her boss' dog was about to give birth to puppies. So, as his dog was one of the breeds on our shortlist, I asked Kirsty to pass a letter on to him saying how interested we were in having one of the pups.

A few days later and on my 50th birthday, my life changed for the better in the most miraculous way. Tony and I had decided to go to a nearby cathedral town for the day to celebrate. As we were driving there, I received a phone call from Kirsty's boss to say the puppies had been born and that he was happy for us to have one of them in eight weeks' time. This was the most amazing news to get on my birthday; a day that had previously been filled with dread due to reaching the age of 50! The second part of this most amazing day was what I'd call a true 'God instance'.

During my first inpatient stay at Forest Field Hospital in 1998 I had met and become friends with another patient called Emily. We became very close but hadn't seen each other since 2000. I was aware from seeing posts on Facebook that, 18 years on, she was still chronically ill with anorexia. I knew that Emily still lived where Tony and I were spending the day and for some reason, on the journey there, I just had this feeling that I was going to bump into her.

An hour or so after arriving Tony and I sat outside the cathedral and who walks by but Emily! She was instantly recognisable because sadly she was terribly emaciated and obviously still seriously unwell. I wasn't sure that she would recognise me after so many years, but Tony encouraged me to go and say hello. I called out her name and she immediately said "Oh my God ... Lily" and we gave each other the biggest hug. I arranged to meet her again a few days later and it was like we had never been apart. We reconnected from where we had left off 18 years previously and quickly became very close again. From that moment on, we chatted or texted most days. What was so miraculous was how we had managed to bump into Emily that day when she was so rarely out of hospital due to her anorexia.

My hope was that I could somehow help Emily recover. She had been ill for so long and had been an inpatient in Eating Disorder

Units many times. I myself was only a little underweight at this time, but that changed once we got our puppy home. Over the following months, the love I felt for our new dog, Sapphire, distracted me from the depressive thoughts I'd had previously and reduced my focus on trying to lose weight at all costs. My depression and anxiety gradually began to lift.

Emily and I helped each other over the next two years. Unfortunately, I wasn't able to help Emily gain weight or change her anorexic behaviour, but I hope I supported her in the best way I could, whether by visiting her in hospital or letting her vent her frustrations out on me. I was growing close to Emily and loved her like a little sister. However, three or four months after reuniting with her, she became really poorly with pneumonia and was admitted to a general hospital. I remember telling Tony that I was scared she was going to die when I had only just reconnected with her: she had become so very special to me. Emily was seriously ill at this time and often told me about dreams / hallucinations she had when her blood sugars kept dropping low. These dreams / visions always had God present, and she would often visit the hospital chapel armed with questions for the vicar to answer.

A few weeks later, Emily was deemed well enough to leave hospital and was transferred to an Eating Disorder Unit in Somerset. The unit was a long way from her home, but at that time it was the only place in the country with an available bed. During her stay there, Emily completed an online Alpha Course via Zoom with the curate from the city's Cathedral. She was from Emily's home-town and they became very close. Three or four months later, she decided she'd like to be Confirmed. Reluctantly, the Unit hospital staff allowed her overnight leave to travel home for the service. As you can imagine, I was chuffed to bits that Emily's faith was growing and I prayed that this could have a truly positive impact on her life.

CHAPTER 17

A Devastating Loss

Sadly Emily was unable to cope whenever she was discharged from hospital and inevitably, within a short time, would be re-admitted. From the time we reconnected it was clear to me that the consultants in the eating disorder units had given up trying to get Emily well and instead only focused on increasing her weight by a few kilos; basically, to keep her alive. Every new hospital admission seemed to make her worse. By now she was completely institutionalised, having been admitted more than 50 times. This, together with being discharged at such low weights and with very little support in the community, meant she had little hope of recovery and a life without anorexia. Emily and I often spoke frankly about her treatment seeming to be merely palliative, but I'm unsure if she ever really understood how ill she was.

During the two years between 2018 and 2020, I would go and visit Emily whenever I could (either when she was in hospital or when she was at home). During the Covid Pandemic this wasn't always possible and instead we would talk on the phone and text almost daily. We were always completely honest with each other, understood each other's difficulties and would often just 'off-load' our frustrations on each other. I always worried that Emily could not go on forever at such a low weight and the fonder I became of her, the more my fear grew of how I'd cope if she died. How on earth would I deal with the loss of Emily, who was by now my closest and dearest friend?

I admit that although I loved Emily dearly, I began to feel increasingly frustrated that I could not help her, or that she wasn't prepared - or able - to change her anorexic behaviour. Although she hated being in hospital and seemed to find each stay more difficult, she always ended up having yet another admission shortly after being discharged. I now recognise the frustrations often experienced by sufferers' family and friends. I shared these frustrations with my sister about a year after I reconnected with Emily. She told me that she used to feel the same way when I was ill. To non-sufferers the solution to anorexia is simple ... "eat more and exercise less". If only it were that simple. No one seems to know how best to treat this awful illness, which is probably why anorexia has the highest death rate among all psychiatric illnesses.

2020 was a particularly difficult year for Emily. She had been admitted back to Forest Field but because of the Pandemic lockdown she wasn't allowed any visits from family or friends. She was not allowed off the unit even for a short period of time. Emily was frustrated with this and incredibly bored, which made her hospitalisation more difficult than ever before.

The final time I saw Emily was after her discharge in October 2020. She asked if I could drive her to the supermarket so that she could stock up on tinned food and non-perishables. As always, we began our time together with a coffee before tackling the shopping. I often wonder what I would have said to her if I had known it would be the last time I saw her?

On 10 November 2020 I had a phone call from Emily, but to my great regret I didn't answer as I was with another friend at the time. However, I sent her a text later that day and then left a voicemail the following morning. It was very unlike her not to respond, so I sent a further two texts asking if she was OK. I heard nothing back. Two days later I was phoned by Emily's mum who tearfully told me that Emily had died. Her poor parents had found her dead in her house. They had gone there because they were worried she hadn't been in contact with them.

Although it seemed inevitable that Emily couldn't go on forever, with years of anorexia taking its toll on her body, her death was still an horrific shock for me and very difficult to come to terms with. I was devastated and didn't know how on earth I'd ever cope without my most dear and trusted friend. We understood each other and connected in a very special way, so much so that she really was the younger sister I never had.

What I have come to realise in the two-and-a-half years or so since Emily's death, is that there is much more to life than being controlled or obsessed by one's weight and body size. So much of life, especially socialising, revolves around food and obsessing over what goes in your mouth leads to a non-existent social life, with a resultant lack of friendships, an increase in isolation and a basic lack of enjoyment. Restricting food, and in my case increasing exercise, led to many damaged relationships - with my family, Tony, work colleagues and friends.

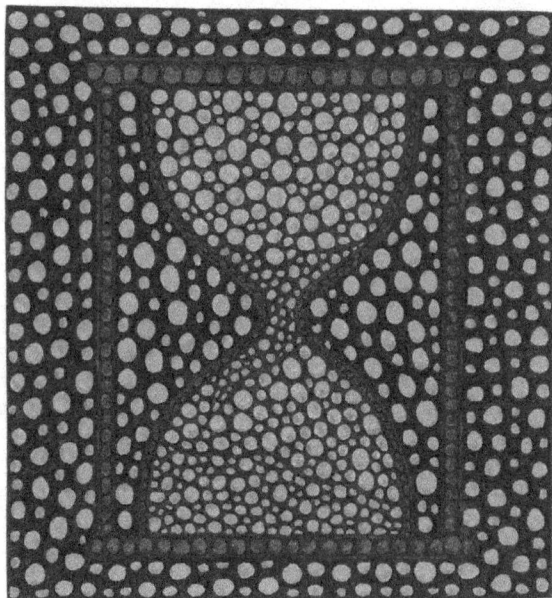

I feel time is running out for me

If Emily had met someone – like I met Tony - then I'm sure her life would have been very different. Unfortunately, she was never well enough to have a boyfriend because her illness always got in the way. My dream for her was to meet a 'life-saver', just as I was fortunate enough to have done with Tony. I have no doubt that Tony saved my life because, without him, I'm sure I wouldn't be here today. He has supported me emotionally, psychologically, socially and financially over the years and shown me that there can be a life without anorexia.

If only Emily had realised what an amazing, clever, loyal and loved person she was. Anorexia destroyed her life, ultimately cutting it short at 39 years old. When she died, she left her family and close friends, including me, distraught. I often wonder whether she ever comprehended just how much she was loved or how her death would affect so many people?

I miss Emily very much. I can't comprehend how many families, carers and friends of sufferers go through this indescribable grief when loved ones are lost to this terrible illness. Even the top eating disorder specialists don't seem to know how best to treat anorexia and bulimia. If they did, then maybe Emily would be still be alive today.

I read some shocking figures recently that were posted on the Instagram account of the eating disorder campaigner Hope Virgo:

* The rate of suicide is 23 times higher in people with eating disorders compared to the general population.
* In the United States 10,200 people die each year because of eating disorders.
* 1 in 5 deaths in eating disorder patients are reported to be taking place because of suicide.

Of course, it is not just suicide that causes death in eating disorder sufferers; often physical causes are to blame, such as heart attacks and pneumonia, but the suicide statistics highlight what a depressive, isolating and overwhelming illness it is. I heard the following quote from a soap opera in which one of the characters had committed suicide - I feel it perfectly sums up how I felt when I tried on a number on occasions to take my own life:

"He didn't commit suicide because he wanted to die …. he was just so desperate he didn't know what else to do".

I have already mentioned the anxiety recovery course that I attended. There, it was explained how important it is to participate in enjoyable activities which distract from obsessive behaviour. Emily was brilliant at attempting to distract herself with arts and crafts, an ambition to learn new things, a love for nature and gardening, and meeting up with close friends. Nevertheless, tragically her anorexia was so deeply entrenched that she was never able to stop the controlling and obsessive behaviour that is inevitable when an eating disorder takes over your life.

CHAPTER 18
The Importance of Hope

Throughout my illness I longed to hear from people who had recovered from anorexia because this would have given me hope that recovery was possible. During all my years of hospital stays and therapy, I never got to meet anyone or even hear of anyone who had recovered so I was never able to believe I could recover. However, I am living proof that there is always hope and hope is essential if sufferers are to keep battling on and to never give up.

While in Forest Field Hospital I read a phrase in a book that I thought was apt for describing how to recover from anorexia. That phrase is: 'the only way out is through.' By writing my story I would like others to realise that you have to go through a lot of awful feelings in order to come out the other side. It is only by travelling through the bad times that you can come out the other side and recover. I so wish that someone had explained this to me during my treatment – I may then not have given up hope on so many occasions.

One of the greatest frustrations I had while ill was that non-sufferers just didn't seem to be able to understand the way I was feeling. They didn't understand why I considered myself fat, why I was having such destructive thoughts, why losing weight was the only thing that mattered to me, why I felt I didn't deserve to eat and most importantly why I was destroying my life in such a way. My hope is that whoever reads this book will gain a greater understanding of why anorexics (or bulimics) do what they do and why they have the thoughts they do. I am aware that each anorexic or bulimic is a different case and what troubled me would not necessarily trouble other sufferers. Nevertheless there will be some similarities and my aim is to open the minds of parents, partners, siblings, friends and health care professionals as to how desperate and destructive the thoughts of sufferers can be.

One of the biggest fears I had with inpatient care was that I would be 'fattened up', only to a reach target weight without any change to the terrible, negative thoughts in my head. For me this fear became a reality in two of my hospital stays. My depression was always worse when I reached target weight and I strongly believe that this is why so many anorexics gain weight in hospital only to lose it all again when they leave. For anorexics, weight gain is so out of their comfort zone that they just do not have the brain capacity to 'work through it.' We know that malnutrition affects the way the brain works, but in my experience even after weight gain the brain doesn't start functioning properly again until sometime after that weight is maintained. This is why I feel so strongly that support needs to continue for a long time after a healthy weight has been achieved and maintained. Unfortunately, due to the lack of NHS funding, there are a limited number of inpatient beds in the country. In addition, help in the community is restricted unless a sufferer is under a certain BMI, but this level is dangerously low, which allows the eating disorder to become entrenched even before treatment can begin.

During the time I was the most unwell, my drawings became the only way I could adequately communicate my thoughts and feelings. Without this outlet for venting my thoughts, I am certain I would not be here telling my story. Not many people saw my drawings, but a few did; my consultant at Forest Field Hospital was adamant that I needed to stop drawing at once, because the drawings were just reinforcing my negative thoughts. I was frustrated with him not understanding why I had done them – first to 'vent' my thoughts in a non-destructive way and second to try to show how I was feeling so that others could understand. A few others in the medical profession said that my drawings did increase their understanding, but after the comment from my consultant I was reluctant to show other people. I understand how my drawings could have been seen as a form of negative reinforcement - and yes, I was obsessed with death and skeletons (as my mum told me in January 2014) - but I found it a tremendous release of my pent-up emotions.

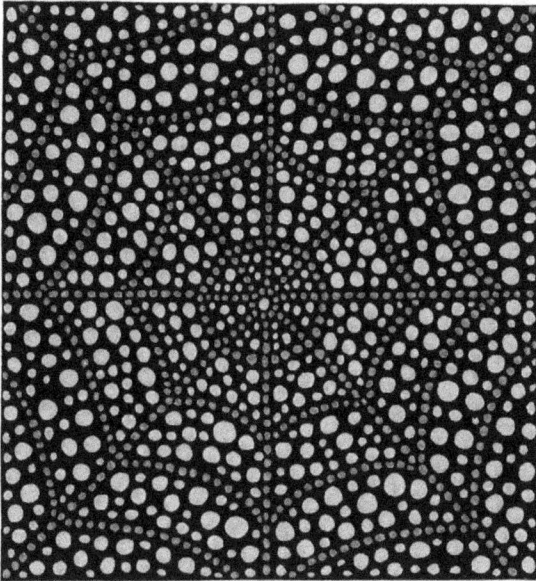

I feel so trapped with my
thoughts and feelings

Over the three or four years that I drew, I had four very distinctive styles. First, I began by copying skeletons and body parts from biology and physiology books. Second, I drew images of how

I planned to kill myself, as well as how I was feeling, but I was always disappointed with these because, although they were expressive, they didn't demonstrate much artistic skill. When I had my second admission to Forest Field Hospital, I began the third style which was founded on an obsession with 'fat globules' taking over my body - so all my drawings were made up of circles (fat globules). When I was admitted to Warren Abbot, the style changed

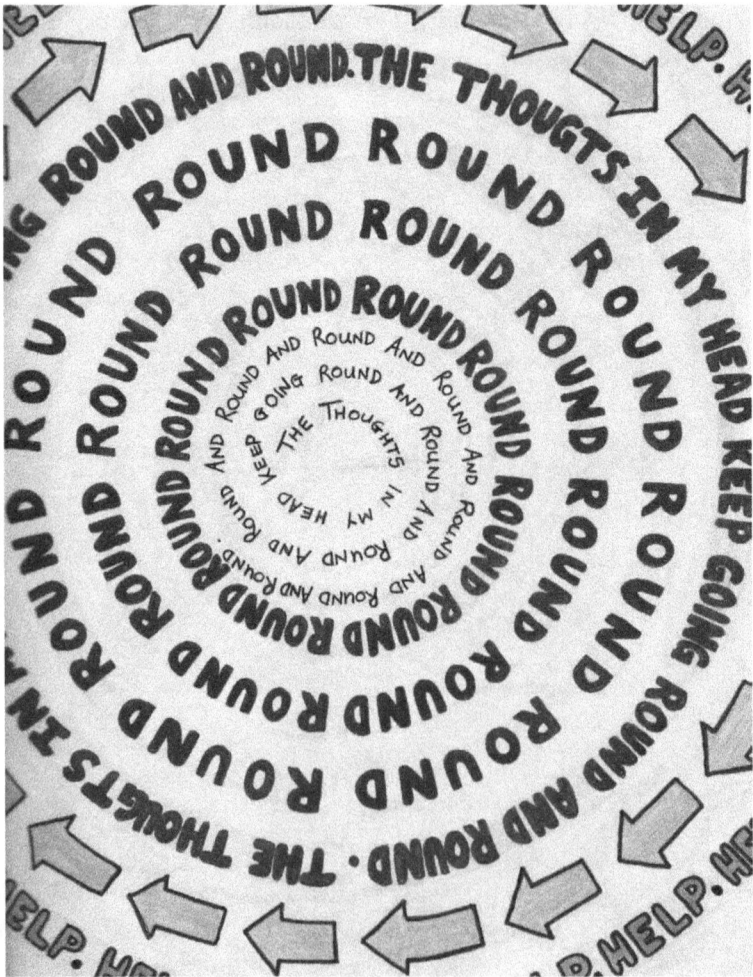

for the fourth time and became a mixture of words and patterns illustrating my thoughts (an example of which you can see opposite).

All four different styles needed various degrees of concentration, skill, and imagination and changed depending on how ill I was. With my first style I initially copied a drawing from an artist and then added a comment about how it was relevant to me, or explained what thoughts I was having at the time. I continued to make comments on my drawings in all four styles, until it almost became a diary of how I was feeling each day.

I learnt recently that my consultant at Forest Field told my parents that he had little doubt I was going to end up killing myself. I honestly believe that if it wasn't for my drawings, I would have attempted suicide more times or caused myself a lot more harm. At times during my illness self-harming, mainly by cutting, became a real problem. For me, self-harm became yet another avenue for 'venting' the destructive and negative thoughts I constantly had. The relief was only ever temporary, but the scars weren't – now, 25 years on, I still have visible scars. They are, in fact, the only physical sign I still have that indicates I had a mental health problem. Even after all this time, these scars still cause me a lot of shame – shame not because of what I went through, but shame because too many people jump to the conclusion that self-harmers are attention seekers.

My scars used to restrict what I wore in the summer and caused me all sorts of embarrassment. For example, in my first knee operation, the anaesthetist asked about my scars while administering a general anaesthetic to me. I had to try and explain what they were, years after I'd stopped cutting. The year before, while teaching PE to primary-school children, I felt I couldn't wear a short-sleeved top, even though it was boiling hot, for fear of the children asking questions about my scars, or them being seen by other teachers. I was frightened I would be sacked for being a bad role-model.

On another occasion, while at a wedding, a friend's husband asked what I had done to get so many scars on my arms and, even though I had never met him before. I had to go through the embarrassment of telling a complete stranger that I used to self-harm.

Some may question why I care what other people think, but unfortunately I am still very concerned about that. Tony quite often tells me that I should be proud of my scars as it shows that I've come from a really bad place to a good one and what an achievement that is. Unfortunately, I seem unable to feel that way.

I felt so desperate while I was cutting myself. I didn't feel I had a future. So when nurses and others said that I would regret scars in later life, it meant nothing.

The most helpful person in my recovery was undoubtedly Tony. When I was really poorly, I wouldn't see him, let alone let him touch me and many times I tried to end our relationship. I had no room in my life for anything other than to diet, exercise and lose weight. However, he refused to finish with me and was always there when I needed him. More than that, though – he never gave up believing that I would get better. Even when my consultant told him that I wasn't going to get better, he refused to accept it. The same consultant also told me that my relationship with Tony wouldn't last - I think he has been proved wrong as we have now been together almost 32 years.

It is important to point out that I still have certain struggles. I still lack self-confidence and worry far too much what other people think of me. I still don't like my body or the way I look. I always seem to think others will judge me if they see 'fat' on my body. I think this stems from thinking that if I'm repulsed by it, then others will feel the same. I have also come to realise that no woman I know is ever entirely happy with their body and would like to alter certain aspects of their figure - and that is probably also the case for many men.

I have also discovered that it is important to include things in one's life that are not only enjoyed, but also give a sense a self-worth. For years I didn't have any self-worth, especially as my illness caused me to resign from my teaching job and not work for such a long time afterwards. I did not feel a valued member of society and constantly had the feeling that I had completely wasted my life. In 2013 I began working for a football club who made me redundant in 2017 and this also had a detrimental effect on my self-worth. However, I really enjoy my present work in social care; a job that has helped my self-worth to improve. The pay is poor but I've learnt that it is much more important to enjoy your job and to feel that you are making a difference.

Getting my dog, Ted, all those years ago was a real source of enjoyment. I strongly feel that Ted looked after me as much as I looked after him. In the early days after discharge from Warren Abbot he gave me something on which to focus and I knew that he relied on me to stay well so that I could look after him. Following my relapse in 2015, getting Sapphire in 2018 and then a second dog – Angus - in 2020 had the same positive impact.

During my childhood I am certain my parents did everything they could to treat my brother, my sister and me the same and everything they did was with our best interests at heart. However, to be treated the same way presumed that we had the same personalities, intelligence etc. I was undoubtedly more sensitive than my brother and sister and would often feel very upset about comments that the other two were able to simply brush off. It has only been relatively recently that people have pointed out to me that being sensitive is not necessarily a negative thing (as I had always been led to believe by Mum and Dad) but a positive personality trait which can, for example, lead to having more empathy for others. However, it's also true to say that being sensitive makes one much more likely to get hurt.

Mum and Dad have mellowed somewhat as they have got older, but I still find it hard to do something if I don't first get their approval, and I still feel deep down that I should do as they say (even at the age of 55). They were always generous with family holidays when we were growing up and today they continue to be generous with their money. However, I still have to try and let hurtful comments pass over my head rather than let them affect me (which at times can be quite a battle). I am such a different personality from my Mum and I think that is why it is always going to be a tricky relationship. My Dad, on the other hand, never shows any emotion; it is always a case of 'stiff upper lip' and so with him too I find it difficult to discuss my feelings or thoughts.

My aim for this book has been to give hope to sufferers of eating disorders who feel it's impossible to recover. Another aim is to give non-sufferers, whether family, friends, carers or health care professionals, an insight into an anorexic's mind, and thus a greater understanding of the type of thoughts that their partner, daughter, son, sibling, friend, or patient may be experiencing - I hope that I have managed to achieve this.

AND FINALLY ...

My ultimate goal while suffering with anorexia was to lose weight at all costs, whether it was to restrict certain foods, over-exercise, purge or obsessively calorie count. This compulsion over-rode everything that was previously important to me and losing weight became my number one focus in life. It took precedence over the risk of losing friends, damaging family relationships and having to give up work. Ultimately my aim was to fade away and disappear from the world I was living in.

As I was recovering from my most recent slip back to anorexic habits (2015-2018) I learnt how important it was to do things that taught me how to laugh again. I couldn't remember the last time I had laughed like I did when I became friends with Kirsty. My friendship with her taught me how to have fun again. I also realised how important it was to identify activities that made me feel good about myself and that don't involve destructive behaviour in order to burn calories or lose weight. I've now realised that I can't do any individual activity / exercise such as swimming or gym workouts without the urge to constantly set targets, or goals to beat my previous performance. I can't seem to just go for a pleasurable swim like others, but instead always seem to overdo it.

Another thing I learnt was to participate in activities that involve making new friends and socialising with them. This meant making friends with others that do not have eating disorders or suffer depression and anxiety. It's important to say that I still have friends that suffer with these conditions; it's just that now I also have friends that do not. I can now have fun and a laugh with friends that are mentally well and so be refreshed enough to offer support to those friends who are sadly not so well. It was once said to me that I need to surround myself with 'radiators' - those that make me feel good - rather than 'drains' - those that sap you of any joy and drag you down to feel depressed like themselves.

We all have times when we feel low but I slowly began to realise that it's not normal to never laugh, not enjoy anything, feel constantly unhappy, obsessed with weight, appearance and food and even suicidal. Having anorexia or bulimia slowly robs you of the person you once were or should be. For me, it made me paranoid, obsessed, angry, suicidal, ritualistic and socially isolated. It was impossible to stop the inner critical voice overcoming and destroying the person I used to be. However, having come out the other side, I now know that there is a life to relish and enjoy, away from anorexia. It's not at all easy but slowly life can return to how it should be. For me, doing things that are fun and that make me laugh slowly outweighed the negative thoughts and feelings that I will probably always feel about myself.

Since I first became ill, it is true to say some treatments have changed, especially with types of therapy and the amount of calories that need to be consumed while in inpatient Eating Disorder Units. However, it is sad to say that the number of adults and children suffering from eating disorders is rising, the funding is reducing and the services offered in the community lacking. It breaks my heart that unless you are so severely underweight and meet the BMI range in which treatment can begin, you seem to be left to suffer on your own. It is well reported that the longer a person has an eating disorder, the harder it is to treat.

There is also the issue of benefits from the Department of Work and Pensions. I know how scared Emily was about losing her benefits if deemed well enough to no longer receive them. This is the same with Georgie, who was one of Emily's closest friends and to whom I have become close since Emily's death. It is terrifying to feel that if you put on weight, you are deemed healthy and so risk financial insecurity because you will no longer receive benefits. Emily worked an hour a day when out of hospital, Georgie works four mornings a week. So, in order to become financially independent a sufferer needs to go from working hardly at all to working full time. This is clearly too big a jump and I am sure that the fear of losing benefits is a major hindrance to recovery.

What helped me to get my life back:

* Knowing / believing that my husband loves me even if I don't know why
* Recognising that no matter what my weight / size I will never be happy with my body or the way I look. Trying to redesign my body is therefore a waste of time and a waste of a life
* Accepting that I need to remain on anti-depressants to stay well
* Taking part in activities that increase my self-worth, self-confidence, happiness and social life
* Giving myself permission to practise self-care activities
* The huge therapeutic effect that getting Sapphire, and then two years after that, Angus, had on my life (our two present dogs).

* Being aware that I see myself in 'remission' from anorexia rather than being 'fully recovered' – understanding that I can't be complacent and think I can control the warning signs of a relapse.
* Having a job that I enjoy is more important than status or salary
* A love of gardening
* Trying to see the positives rather than the negatives.
* Accepting that I need to stay away from individual sports (such as swimming or gym workouts) as I seem incapable of controlling/competing against my previous times or distances
* Starting to play a new sport called Pickleball, which has had the added bonus of making great new friends, having many laughs, enjoying the social side, the chance of playing at a reasonable level and of improving as a player. I am forever indebted to Pippa and Ivan for introducing me to this most fabulous sport in 2021 and becoming two of my dearest friends
* I fully believe that God helped me through my battle with anorexia and I recommend anyone to reach out to Him for help – possibly, like me, through an Alpha Course.

*****

APPENDICES 1 and 2

The songs that Tony wrote that became so important to me

If You Call His Name

If you call His name, if you seek His power,
He will light your way in your darkness hour,
And if you touch His cloak just gently,
He will turn His face to you,
He will smile and say "I love you,
And I know what you've been through.
Oh precious child, oh precious one,
How I have waited for you to come
To me."

I know that you feel that all is lost,
Your pain's so great, it is all hopeless,
But if you touch His hands just gently,
You will know He has scars too,
And He will say "Yes I have suffered,
I have cried out just like you.
Oh precious child, oh precious one,
You will find peace when you come
To me."

I know you think this can't be true,
How could He love someone like you,
But if you touch The Cross just gently,
His tears on you will fall,

And He will whisper "I do love you,
I am giving you my all.
Oh precious child, oh precious one,
I die so that you can become
Set free."

I know it's hard to take this in,
That all your wrongs have been laid on Him,
Yet this gift He offers gently,
Longing for you to accept,
So He can say "My child you're safe now,
I am your saviour, I'm your strength.
Yes precious child, yes precious one,
Your past is dead, new life's begun
With me."

Out of the Depths

Out of the depths I cry out to You, oh Lord,
Won't You please hear me, do not hide Your face,
My soul is in anguish, it pleads "Why oh why Lord?"
I'm worn out from groaning, I'm drenched in my tears,
Sorrow pervades me, Lord please don't forsake me,
For You are my comfort, You are my strength.

Save me with Your unfailing love,
All my hope rests in Your hand,
I put my trust in You, my Rock,
Though so much I do not understand.

As the heavens are higher than the earth,
So Your ways are higher than my own,
Lord in Your mercy please draw near,
Do not let me walk alone.

Yours is an unfailing love,
Lord, I reach out for Your hand,
Embraced in Your arms I know,
For I know that You are good
That one day I will understand.

Taken from Psalms 6 and 130 and Isaiah 55

APPENDIX 3

The Testimony I Read Out at my Baptism

"At the age of 17, I developed anorexia and only recovered from it 22 years later, after spending a great deal of time in hospital. During this time I still managed to go to university and I taught for seven years at a school, which is where I met Tony. However during my worst times I felt I didn't want to live anymore and tried to commit suicide three times. I was in a bad way. Despite the opinions of my psychiatrists, Tony stuck by me throughout.

However, four years ago I slowly began putting on weight. This was not a conscious decision but I seemed to lose all the willpower I had had to starve myself. I now believe that as so many people had been praying for me, God was enabling me to eat again and to no longer wish to die. At this time, Tony asked me to marry him, and I was able to see a future for myself.

So six months before our wedding, I did an Alpha Course at the local Free Church. The Alpha Course is an introduction to Christianity, which I can really recommend. However, I did this course more to please Tony than anything else. But I did make the decision to ask Jesus into my life at this time. I felt a tingling sensation when I said the prayer, but it wasn't as if the heavens opened. Nevertheless, looking back I realise that my life started to change for the better from that point. We joined a home group at the Free Church, and I began to read the Bible and generally tried to get closer to God.

In August 2008 Tony and I got married. Leading up to it, I was a nervous wreck. So many people were at our wedding and I had always hated being centre of attention. I was so anxious I didn't think I would even make it down the aisle without having a panic attack. I arrived at the church and it was pouring with rain and really windy. All of a sudden a man met me at the car with a golfing umbrella in hand. I thought what a lovely, thoughtful, kind person and was really moved by the gesture … anyway walking down the aisle, not only did I feel like a princess but I have never felt so confident. The service was amazing and moved many people (including me). I now realise this was down to the power of prayer.

I became even more convinced that there is something in this 'God thing' so I started going regularly to church. One year later I got pregnant but unfortunately had a miscarriage. I remember blaming God and thinking "you've helped me so much in the last two years so why haven't you allowed me to have a baby?" I stopped going to church for a while and then began to think, well maybe God made it happen for a reason. I'm beginning to realise that we need to trust God even if we don't understand the reasons why. So I started going to church again.

Then the vicar asked Tony and I if we would help out on the Alpha Course last September (2010). I thought "how can I do that? I don't know much about God so what could I possibly offer?" and also I'm not very confident with people. However reluctantly I decided to give it a try. As the course progressed, I learnt so much and met someone who is now my dear friend. She allayed my fears of not being good enough to help out, and always said and prayed real words of encouragement. From this Alpha course 'The Way' home group was formed, which is full of people I love to bits.

I then started to go to the 6.30pm service every week, where I love the worship and get so much out of the sermons. I always feel close to God at this service, so as I began to increase my faith I started to think about reaffirming my baptism vows, making an outward sign that I am serious about God. I have wanted to do this for a while but didn't feel happy about it while I was still smoking. Smoking was an addiction left over from my anorexic days where I smoked to control my hunger. The longest I had gone without a cigarette in 21 years was 12 days. I told my dear Christian friend I met on the Alpha course, the guilt I felt at smoking while being a Christian, and I have since found out she prayed for me ever since that conversation. So one day I decided to put all my trust in God and every time I had a craving for a cigarette I prayed to Him that I would get strength from Him to overcome it. I kept thinking of the verse in 1 Corinthians Ch10 v13 .. "And God is faithful; He will not let you be tempted beyond what you can bear." I have now gone 10 weeks without a cigarette and am trusting in God that I won't ever smoke again.

I believe God has done so much for me. He has allowed me to recover from anorexia and depression and saved my life at least three times. Also He has allowed me to be very happily married. This is why I want to show my commitment to God by reaffirming my baptism vows".

-